Intermittent Fasting:

Guide for women and men: lose weight or build muscle for men and women + 14 day meal plan for weight loss

Tim Martin

Additionally, the information in the following pages is intended only for informational purposes and should thus be thought of as universal. As befitting its nature, it is presented without assurance regarding its prolonged validity or interim quality. Trademarks that are mentioned are done without written consent and can in no way be considered an endorsement from the trademark holder.

Table of Contents

Introduction

Congratulations for your copy of *Intermittent Fasting: Guide for Women and Men*! We are very excited for you to use this resource to aid your journey with intermittent fasting.

You've heard the hype about intermittent fasting and people getting results without stressing over following a diet or doing 18 hours of cardio a week and now you want to give it a shot and see for yourself. Well, we're here to help you get started. In this book, you will find the knowledge you need to implement fasting into your lifestyle. You will learn how long humans have been using fasting for health and many other reasons. Then you'll find the explanation for how fasting can help YOU drop weight and why it is effective. You'll learn the health benefits you can reap and the potential risks you might encounter. Then we'll highlight the different methods you can choose from and what each entails so you can work out the type of fasting is right for you. Whether you are looking to gain muscle or lose weight, you'll find tips and tricks to help you get the results you want faster. As a bonus to get you started, this book also contains a 14-day healthy eating meal plan following the 5:2 method and an introduction to meal prep to make your lifestyle stress-free!

There are plenty of books on intermittent fasting on the market, we are thankful that you chose this one! Every effort was made to ensure it is full of as much useful information as possible, and we hope you enjoy!

Chapter 1: A Brief History of Fasting

Fasting has been used for many purposes across many cultures even before written history. It has been used for religious reasons, protests, medicinal cures, and rituals. In religions, from Paganism to Catholicism, people fast to worship or to observe holy days. In the animal kingdom, many organisms fast when they are ill or stressed. Understanding the historical significance of fasting can help illustrate the benefits it brings about. Many people in modern times are skeptical about using fasting for health purposes because there has not been a sufficient amount of research to prove its benefits. However, history shows many cultures who incorporated fasting for similar purposes despite not having interactions with each other.

Nearly every major religion practices fasting for various spiritual reasons. Muslims fast during the holy month of Ramadan and Catholics fast during Lent. Judaism has its own occasions of fasting, including Yom Kippur. Hinduism, Paganism, Gnosticism, Christianity, Wicca, etc. Religions incorporate fasting in various degrees for spiritual reasons. Even Native Americans used fasting to please their deities. Religious purposes for fasting usually include an element of sacrifice or penance, but also involve elements of purification, spiritual visions, and mourning. Some primitive societies used fasting as a ritual in coming-of-age ceremonies. Many times, fasting is for spiritual purposes because they believe it breaks the attachment to food that can impede our ability to focus on more beneficial things. Rather than feeding the body, the focus shifts to feeding the mind and spirit.

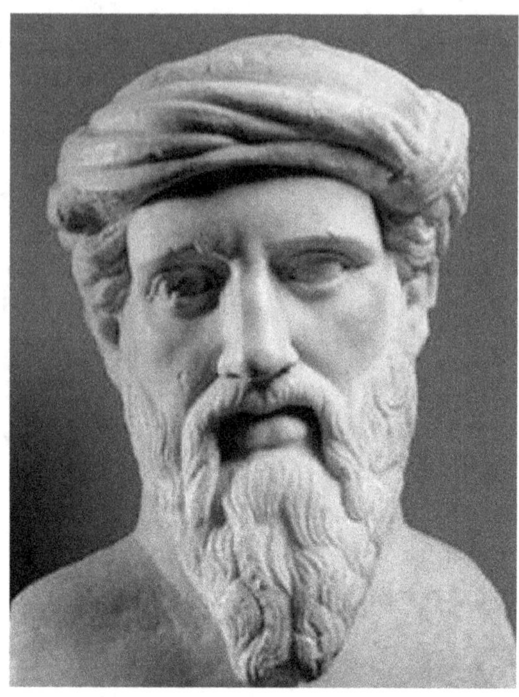

The Greek philosopher and mathematician Pythagoras in the years of 570 to 500 BC is known to have praised the effects of fasting. In his late 30s, Pythagoras wanted to join a school of mysticism at a temple called Diospolis in Egypt but was told that he could not be allowed entry until he had fasted for 40 days and practice a specific breathing pattern. He initially did not want to do this, but after finding no other ways to be accepted in this school, he completed the 40-day rite of passage. By the end of the fast, he proclaimed that he had been purified and was now more in touch with his existence. He said he was a new man, and that truth was now more than a concept. It was life. Afterward, he incorporated fasting into his life and praised its virtues. He was even known to have required his followers and disciples to fast for a duration of 40 days consuming only water to improve their mental clarity and creativity. His followers also practiced a strict vegetarian diet when not fasting, but did not consume beans.

Another famous Greek figure, the physician Hippocrates advised fasting to his patients because according to him, the human body "carries within him a doctor" and fasting helps that doctor do his work.

In the middle ages, there are accounts of aristocrats who frequently indulged in food and drink in excess. One particular man by the name of Luigi Di Cornaro, born in the year 1465, partook of this lifestyle. By the age of 40, he was bedridden with illness. Doctors throughout Italy attempted to cure him, but his illness proved to be stubborn. One doctor proposed a treatment that went against the medical opinions of the time: fasting. Cornaro implemented this concept of periodic fasting and survived what was thought to be a terminal illness. Not only did he survive, but over time his illnesses subsided completely. After being thought near death in his 40s, Luigi Di Cornaro lived to be 104 years old.

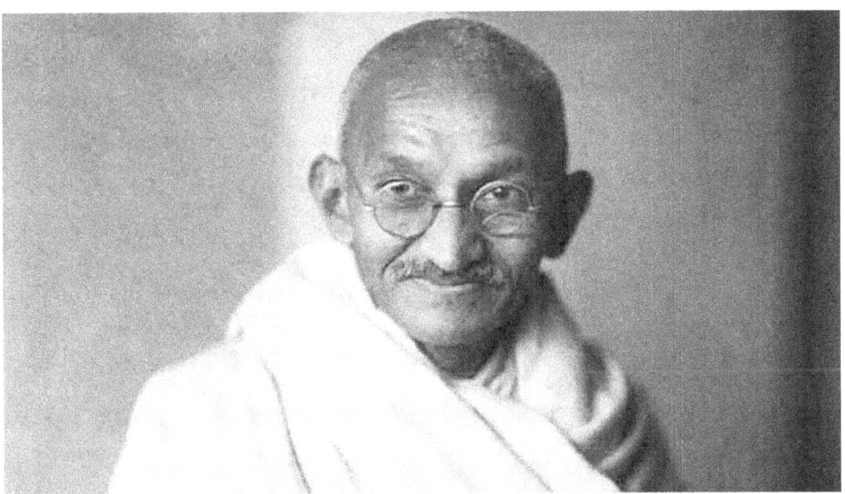

Mohandas Karamchand Gandhi, or Mahatma Gandhi as he is commonly known, fasted 17 times during India's freedom movement. Gandhi used fasting as a form of nonviolent protest. He was an iconic embodiment of the belief that humans are capable of compassion and tolerance, and that all are good at heart. He began fasting to atone for the sins of others and to mourn those lost to injustices. He later fasted during various times of social reform in India. 17 hunger strikes of varying lengths marked Gandhi's life as a leader who believed in humanity and inspired social reform. The longest of these fasts lasted 3 full weeks.

Historically, fasting has always been present in many aspects of culture. During the 19th and 20th centuries, a movement of "natural health practices" in the United States, the United Kingdom, and Germany involved centers where people would go on individually tailored and monitored fasts to treat headaches, allergies, digestive problems, high blood pressure, heart disease and obesity. Treatments last days or involve intermittent fasting techniques for up to 3 months. In the 1920s and 1930s, a doctor in Texas ran a "Health School" where he claimed to have assisted 40,000 patients with recoveries from various illnesses using water fasts. Around the same time, natural health centers also became popular in the United Kingdom, starting in Edinburgh, Scotland and spreading from there. This movement fell off in many areas but is still popular in areas of Europe including Germany, Austria, the Czech Republic, and Hungary.

Fasting is not a new concept, it has been shown in a new light with its rise to stardom in the modern health and fitness community. Since the early 2000s, fitness gurus and everyday Joe's have rediscovered the benefits of incorporating fasting into their health and weight loss journey. The scientific community has only in recent years begun researching the benefits and pitfalls of fasting, so the world of Western medicine does not largely recommend it, but many studies recognize the positive impacts fasting can have on health.

Chapter 2: How and Why Fasting Works

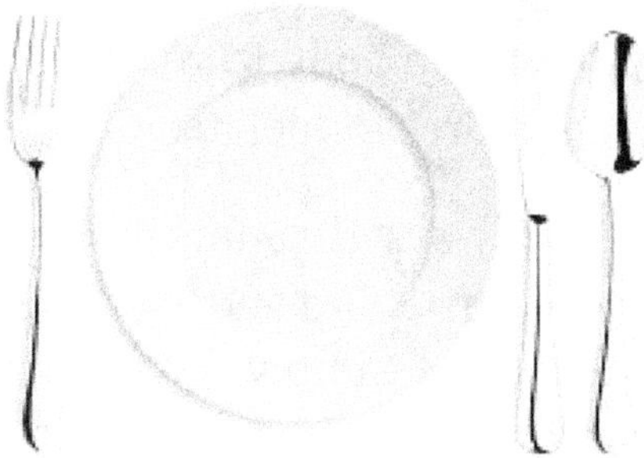

There are various methods of intermittent fasting, so there is bound to be a method that suits your lifestyle. Some methods are more intense than others, and it is to be noted that the fasts that yield more radical results are generally the fasts that require more unreserved dedication. However, even small fasts can boost your metabolism and show positive results. Some methods, like the 5:2 diet, do not require a full fast, but rather a large decrease in the number of calories consumed

Intermittent fasting has become an increasingly popular weight loss tool. In fact, intermittent fasting is the diet of all diets because it isn't a diet at all, it's just a structured eating pattern. The name "intermittent fasting" refers to the practice of consuming calories during a small period of time and avoiding food for a longer duration. On a normal, three-meal-a-day diet, the body is in a "fed" state for the majority of the day. The fed state is when the body is either consuming or digesting food, and during this period the body is utilizing the nutrients for energy. When the fed phase is over, the body goes into a "fasted" state. Having used the energy from the food, it now needs a new source of fuel. On an average diet, this fasted state does not last long enough to allow the body to begin burning fat as fuel because you are providing it with constant caloric intake. This is where intermittent fasting works. By skipping the first meal of the day, fasting for a full 24 hours or by drastically reducing the number of calories for a few days out of the week, fasting allows the body to reach a caloric deficit and start feeding on its fat stores to fuel itself.

While there are a few ways that intermittent fasting aids in weight loss, the most basic and most effective component of the lifestyle is that fasting simply cuts down the number of calories to are eating. Calories are essentially the units of energy that are present in the food we eat. The energy, or calories, in the things we consume fuel the processes that keep our bodies going. When we eat more calories than we need for these processes, the body stores the extra energy in case it needs fuel when it isn't fed. This is an important way the body can protect itself in times of starvation, but when the body does not enter a state of fasting, the energy stores start to build up. This is how we end up gaining more fat than we might prefer to have. If you are looking to lose this fat, the best way is to cut calories and allow the body to use the fuel it has saved up. Many people try low-calorie diets, which can be effective, but they end up frustrated or stressed about counting calories. Depending on which method of intermittent fasting you choose to employ, you may not need to pay attention to calories at all. By fasting for 16 hours a day, you take away one meal and probably a few snacks as well. By fasting for a full 24 hours even once or twice a week, you can subtract thousands of calories from your diet. Of course, depending on your goal, you can alter your calories during your fed window to change how your body responds to intermittent fasting overall.

Other ways fasting stimulates weight loss is through bringing the body into the state of ketosis. The body has two sources from which it can get fuel: sugars and fats. Normally, it gets its energy from sugars that come from the breakdown of carbohydrates. In a carb-heavy diet, the energy is frequently replenished, and the unused energy is stored as fat. An imagery for the use of sugars versus the use of fats is to think of your energy as money in a bank. The fats are money that is locked away in a secure vault. You continually add to this fund, so you have it available when it's needed. The sugars are money that is in your checking account. You have a debit card for this account, so you have access to these funds regularly. Normally, your checking account is filled up with the money you need and then some. So you use what you need and send the extra to your vaulted savings. You can only use one account at a time and accessing your checking account is easy and reliable, so you do not need to go through the hassle of going to the bank and passing the security measures to withdraw from the vault. When your checking account runs dry, you tap into your stored funds. In the same way, the body can also use fats for energy, but it can't use both sugars and fats for fuel at the same time so it will keep them in storage until it has no other choice.

It's unlikely that the body will enter the metabolic state of ketosis within a short time of fasting, but a fast that lasts longer than 24 hours can have this effect. When no sugar is being supplied to the body, it switches into ketosis to get energy. The liver breaks down fat to produce ketone bodies that can be used as fuel in place of sugar.

Some types of cells in the body cannot be fueled by ketones, so these are fed with the glycogen that is stored in the liver or muscles. If the glycogen stores are depleted, new sugars can be made during a process called gluconeogenesis. Protein is a primary component used in this process, which leads many people to be concerned that they will lose muscle mass. Using autophagy, the body actually clears out dead, unnecessary, or worn-out cells which are then used in gluconeogenesis, as well as using proteins from the skin and connective tissue. This can be beneficial to the body because the proteins that are broken down are then replaced. By clearing out the old, it makes way for the new. This can improve cellular function overall. If the body is starved for drastically extended time, it may start to break muscle tissues down. However, on a schedule like in the intermittent fasting methods presented in this book, it is highly unlikely.

As mentioned before, the body cannot run on fats and sugars at the same time. When you break your fast with a normal meal, your body will come out of ketosis and begin to use the sugars in your food for energy. A diet that works well in conjunction with intermittent fasting is the Ketogenic diet. This type of eating focuses on entering and maintaining the metabolic state of ketosis by drastically reducing the number of sugars and carbohydrates intake and focusing heavily on feeding the body healthy fats. If you incorporate this type of meal plan with your fasting routine, you will reap the benefits of ketosis even after breaking your fast. This can yield greater weight loss and muscle gain.

Intermittent fasting is also effective because it can decrease the number of calories you eat even during your fed hours. People who practice fasting consistently for an extended period tend to feel less hungry and get full faster. A hunger hormone called ghrelin stimulates the desire to eat. On a normal eating schedule, this hormone is least present in the morning after waking and spikes around times that people generally eat. If no food is consumed during these spikes, the hormone will decrease, and the urge to eat will pass. After a few days of fasting, the levels of ghrelin in the body start to decrease, even at times when they would normally be higher. In general, the hunger hormone is present in higher levels in women than it is in men. Through fasting, women have a larger drop in ghrelin levels than men do. However, the female body reacts differently to prolonged fasting than the male body does, so it's important for women to be aware of the risks associated with fasting for longer periods of time. Overall, the less you eat, the less hungry you are, so fasting trains the body to not only reduce calories by avoiding meals but to also reduce calories by consuming less during eating.

The presence of the human growth hormone (or HGH) is also increased over a prolonged practice of fasting. HGH has been used since the 1980s by bodybuilders and extreme athletes looking to develop bigger, more toned muscles. In the process of autophagy mentioned earlier in this chapter, excess or damaged parts of the cells are cleared out to make way for healthy cells. The human growth hormone is responsible for completing the cycle of cellular renewal by stimulating the growth of the new healthy muscles. This hormone is also useful in protecting muscle mass and bone density from deteriorating and helping the body to utilize fat during ketosis. HGH is naturally present in the body, usually at its highest levels during sleep and in the morning after waking. With consistent fasting, the levels of HGH rise. This increase is not only present during times when HGH is increased but also during the entire duration of the day. Eating suppresses the human growth hormone, so the longer you fast, the longer you reap the benefits. Note however that it can be dangerous to have extremely high levels of this hormone in the body, so fasting is not advised for individuals with a predisposition to high HGH levels, but in healthy people with normal hormone levels, it is unlikely that fasting will stimulate HGH to produce in dangerous amounts.

The metabolism is also increased through fasting. Some people fear that fasting will cause their body's metabolism to slow down to conserve energy, but actually, the opposite occurs. You may be familiar with the phrase "adrenaline rush" referring to when the body has increased capabilities in times of over-excitement, stress, or danger. Noradrenaline or norepinephrine is the hormone responsible for the increased alertness, heart rate, blood pressure and energy that come with the "fight or flight" response. It increases anxiety, restlessness, and arousal. It also helps form and access memories. Besides enhancing mental and physical abilities, this chemical is helpful in releasing glucose from the glycogen stores in the liver and muscles. This helps the body enter ketosis faster and improves the body's ability to use up the stored glucose. Then, it allows the new glucose to be properly metabolized when you eat. When you fast consistently, levels of noradrenaline in the body rise. This stimulates the metabolism by anywhere from 3.6 percent to 14 percent. Some theorize that this is a biological response that would allow us the energy to seek out food if we were in a starvation state although this has not been proven.

While low-calorie diets are shown to have similar weight loss effects as intermittent fasting, many of these hormonal changes that stimulate weight loss and other health benefits are not present in individuals who practice a calorie-restricted diet that does not involve fasting. Individuals who fast also tend to keep more muscle mass. By improving the function of cells, changing hormone levels, lowering calorie intake, and helping the body burn fat, intermittent fasting helps people lose weight effectively and provides a host of other potential health benefits. It is also more reliably maintainable over a longer period than a non-fasting calorie-restricted diet.

Chapter 3: Health Benefits and Potential Risks

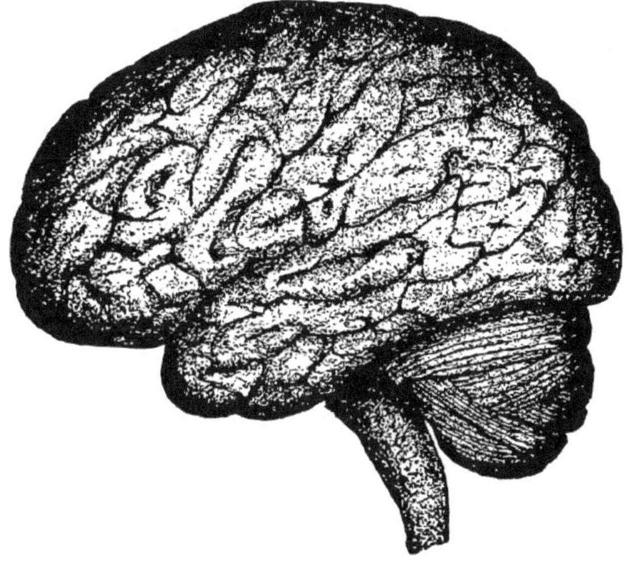

The health benefits of fasting have been proclaimed for millennia by some of the most well-respected doctors and scholars in history. Humans and animals alike have a natural, biological urge to fast when we are sick because our body knows how to heal itself. When it does not have to use so much energy for digesting and absorbing the nutrients in food, the body can focus on fixing the issue. As recently as the 1900s, the medical benefits of fasting have been widely known and appreciated. However, the rise of modern medicine lessened the focus on natural healing methods, and the awareness of fasting and its benefits died down until the early 2000s. Intermittent fasting has gained popularity in the wellness world over the past couple of decades as a wide range of benefits have been reported in both men and women alike. Many people report having lost weight or gained muscle without having changed their overall calorie intake. Others report an increase in energy levels and better sleep. These basic health benefits are clear and appreciated, but intermittent fasting provides even more important health benefits that have led many people to incorporate fasting into their lives long term. From better heart health, boosted brain health, and improved insulin sensitivity to a possibility of cancer prevention, fasting is showing to be a key player in maintaining a healthy body. Research is still being done, but fasting show promise in many areas of health improvement far beyond simple weight loss.

High blood pressure and high cholesterol are both linked to heart disease are concerns for many people. Interestingly, both issues can be improved through fasting. Losing weight, even in small amounts such as 5 pounds, lowers blood pressure. According to one study, people following an intermittent fasting diet reduced their systolic blood pressure up to 11% more than a similar group who followed a normal calorie restrictive diet for the same period. Even when similar amounts of weight were lost in both groups, the other health benefits enjoyed by the intermittent fasting group did not translate in the calorie restricted group.

Cholesterol can also be lowered through intermittent fasting. When you eat too many carbohydrates, your insulin levels will increase. In response to the insulin production, the liver produces more triglycerides. Triglycerides compose half of the bad cholesterol also called VLDL. VLDLs can cause inflammation, damage to arteries, which can lead to several heart complications. By fasting, you lower the insulin levels in your blood which therefore lowers the triglyceride production in the liver. This brings down the levels of bad cholesterol in your body, reduces inflammation, and protects your arteries. All of this happens without damaging the levels of LDLs or good cholesterol in the body which is important for many of the body's hormones and its ability to heal.

Lowering your insulin levels helps lower cholesterol. It also provides other benefits to the body. Insulin is a hormone that sends sugars to the liver and muscles as glycogen to fuel cells and stores unused sugars in fat cells. Over time, a carbohydrate-heavy diet increases insulin levels. The body becomes resistant to insulin, and it loses its efficiency. More insulin is needed to process the sugars it is taking in. Increased insulin levels negatively affect the heart, bones, and pancreas, and can even cause type 2 diabetes. Fasting lowers insulin levels and depletes sugar stores, allowing the body to require less insulin to maintain blood sugar, therefore increasing insulin sensitivity.

Type 2 diabetes is a health condition in which insulin resistance causes blood sugar levels to get dangerously high. If you have type 2 diabetes, fasting has the potential to be incredibly beneficial to your health. Some people suffering from diabetes find that combining intermittent fasting with a ketogenic diet can not only improve blood sugar levels but can even bring them consistently within the normal range. This is not substantiated because research on using fasting as a treatment for diabetes is still in the early stages.

The ketogenic diet and fasting work well together by lowering the number of sugars the body is fed and also allowing the body to use fat for fuel when it is in ketosis. This can lower blood sugar and increase insulin sensitivity to allow the body to process sugars more efficiently. Some diabetics who incorporate fasting and keto foods find that after some time they are able to control their diabetes without medication. It is important to consult your doctor before beginning a fasting routine if you are diabetic, especially if you are on medications that lower your blood sugar because fasting with these medications can lead to dangerously low blood sugar. Some doctors do not recommend intermittent fasting because of the blood sugar fluctuation that comes with it. When skipping meals, the blood sugar will naturally be lower. Then, when you break your fast, the blood sugar will spike. With diabetes, it is ideal to maintain stable blood glucose levels throughout the day. Note that the best fasting results for type 2 diabetes happen in conjunction with a keto diet.

Keto diet in itself has risks for people with diabetes. An overproduction of ketones in ketosis can lead to a condition called diabetic ketoacidosis. This complication can cause complications and can be very severe and dangerous. If you practice fasting and/or a ketogenic diet for the purpose of inducing ketosis, it is important, to talk to your doctor and to monitor your ketone levels closely.

Skipping meals can lead to a negative impact on food choices and may increase your chances of choosing foods that adversely affect your blood sugar. If you do stick with a healthy diet and fasting schedule, you may very well see positive results in weight loss and improvement in insulin sensitivity.

Another risk is that following a fasting routine may increase your chances of gaining back weight should you choose to cease following this routine. Gaining back the weight loss can have a negative effect on insulin levels and lead to complications of diabetes. To summarize, diabetics can benefit from intermittent fasting in certain cases, but the risks associated with this are very high, so it is important to always consult your doctor and figure out the plan that best suits your individual needs.

Your brain can also benefit from fasting. Some studies show that intermittent fasting keeps your brain younger by improving your ability to think, creating new nerve and brain cells, and protecting against degenerative diseases and the effects of a stroke. This research is not definitive, but many studies show promise regarding the effects of fasting on brain health. Fasting increases the rates at which the brain produces new cells in a process called neurogenesis. It also increases the production of a protein in the brain called brain-derived neurotrophic factor, or BDNF, by 50 percent to 200 percent. This protein is a growth protein that is crucial to many aspects of brain function. BDNF not only protects the neurons that you already have but it also allows your brain to produce new neurons and stimulates the connections between them. This allows communication between brain cells to improve which enhances cognitive ability as well as improving your mood and resistance to stress. BDNF is a huge asset to the brain and increased brain capacity is a great benefit of intermittent fasting.

Fasting also increases the production of the human growth hormone (HGH) in the body. HGH is an anabolic hormone that builds muscle and protects you from muscle and bone density loss. It's also anti-aging, so it keeps your body from aging rapidly and increases fat burning. HGH is usually produced during sleep and in the morning after waking, but it is suppressed with the body is fed. During fasting, HGH is released continuously in small amounts during the fasting period. A five day fast can increase human growth hormone levels by as much as 300 percent. This is enough to increase the muscular benefits of the human growth hormone without the side effects of too much. HGH also protects brain health and performance and can positively affect neurogenesis and cognition. During the cell renewal cycle (which is also stimulated by fasting) old, shoddy cells are cleared out to make space for new, healthy cells. HGH helps in rounding out the cycle by stimulating the growth of these healthy cells.

Both the human growth hormone and the brain-derived neurotrophic factor (HGH and BDNF) have anti-aging properties. Studies show that fasting can slow the aging of the brain and protect your body from the negative effects of aging as well. It also is shown to keep the body young at a cellular level by keeping the mitochondria in a state of homeostasis. This basically means that the powerhouses that are processing the energy for your cells are not aging. If the mitochondria do not operate well, your cells will not do their jobs as well, and you age faster.

Intermittent fasting also stimulates a process called autophagy. This process occurs when cells that are not working as well are cleared out and replaced with new ones. Basically, the body tunes up your cells to keep them in good shape. This process can reduce inflammation, help you grow muscle, improve brain function, and help you heal injuries. All around, autophagy allows your body to clear out the junk and make way for the good. During a process called gluconeogenesis which literally means "making new glucose," the body can turn these unnecessary pieces into fuel. Although there is not enough evidence to substantiate the claims, fasting has shown, in some cases, to improve reactions to chemotherapy in cancer patients. One study showed that patients who fasted for 72 hours before undergoing chemotherapy had less damage to the immune system. This is thought to be because the process of autophagy cleared out the immune cells that had been damaged from past chemo treatments and allowed the body to create newer, healthier cells.

Changing your eating schedule can carry plenty of health benefits, but there are also some potential risks that should be taken into consideration before you implement any changes to your lifestyle. Once your body becomes accustomed to alternating between a fasted and fed state, you can start to lose touch with your "hungry" and "full" senses. Because you are either running on low levels of calories, if any or filling yourself up to meet your calorie needs, you may stop paying attention when your body feels hungry or when it's full. This can lead to binge eating and weight gain if you stop intermittent fasting. It is also important to pay attention to your water intake. When starting out with fasting, many people get dehydrated. This can cause headaches and irritability, which can increase stress when coupled with hunger, as well as health issues.

Intermittent fasting presents more health risks in women than it does in men. As women enter the fasted state, their bodies are more inclined to go into starvation mode and try to protect themselves. The natural biological response is to protect the part of the body that could be housing a potential baby. Women have more kisspeptin neurons than men, and these neurons are responsible for stimulating the production of reproductive hormones. Kisspeptin responds to insulin levels and hunger hormones like ghrelin which is also present in higher levels in women. This may be a reason why women are likely to enter starvation mode more quickly than men. The female body alters its reproductive hormones to accommodate the lack of food, and when hormone levels change, the entire body is affected. Prolonged fasting windows can lead to difficulty sleeping, depression and anxiety, as well as fertility issues, shrinkage of the ovaries, and a change in regularity of periods or complete loss of periods altogether. Long-term fasting can even cause early onset menopause. This does not mean that women can't practice intermittent fasting, but it does limit the types of fasting they should practice. The best methods for women involve a 12 to 16-hour fasting window. Although women may fast longer than 16 hours if they desire, anything more than 24 hours will be very hard on the body. Methods like the 5:2 diet that never requires a complete lack of calories is ideal, although methods involve no calorie consumption during the fasting window, such as the 16:8 method, have shown to have better weight loss results in women. A doctor can help you choose a method that is right for you depending on your current health and desired results.

Research to understand the entirety of the benefits and risks associated with intermittent fasting is still in its young stages. However, the diet has gained popularity because the benefits are commonly recognized by the people who practice it. Some studies that have been done on these fasting schedules have compared a group of individuals practicing intermittent fasting with a group that does not fast but does follow a calorie-restricted diet. These studies have found that the amount of weight loss in both groups was similar enough that intermittent fasting could not be found to be a superior weight loss method, but the other hormonal benefits enjoyed by the fasted group did not occur in the calorie restricted group. Overall, each individual will react differently to different methods. Thankfully, intermittent fasting is an umbrella term for various methods of scheduled eating that encompasses something for everyone.

Chapter 4: Circadian Rhythm and Gut Health

Our body has an internal clock of sorts, in the brain that tells our organs how to function based on a 24 hour light and dark cycle. This is called a circadian clock, it maintains a cycle called the circadian rhythm. The circadian clock tells our food processing organs to kick into action around the times when the body normally expects to eat. It also stimulates the levels of energy molecules that tell us to be awake during the day and to sleep at night. Humans are biologically designed to be awake and active during the day and sleep when it's dark. This may stem from prehistoric times when the only light available by which people could perform daily functions was sunlight, so we didn't have many options to eat or work at night. In areas of the world, such as Alaska, the summer months yield up to 19 hours of daylight, and the winter months can seem to be constant darkness. People who live in these areas can experience trouble sleeping at night during the summer and trouble maintaining energy levels during the dark winter days. These types of circadian disruptions can affect many aspects of overall health.

Our metabolism and other processes operate in conjunction with our circadian rhythm, but certain stimuli can confuse our systems. In the evening, the body is more insulin resistant. If we eat in the evening, our blood sugar and insulin levels will increase, and it will take longer for them to return to normal levels. This type of stimulus, as well as others, is called a zeitgeber. Zeitgebers that conflicts with the circadian clock include light, temperature, social cues, food, and drugs. When these are introduced to the body at times that are incongruent with the biological cycle, the body compensates in ways it is not normal. The body tries to maintain the necessary actions to process these stimuli, but this confuses the entire cycle, and it can be difficult to undo it.

A disruption in the circadian rhythm can cause metabolic problems such as prediabetes, elevated blood sugar, and insulin resistance. These issues can lead to weight gain and inefficient absorption of nutrients from food. People who work night shifts or experience insomnia are more likely to have health issues associated with metabolic dysfunction. Cortisol and blood pressure levels can rise, as well as lowering the levels of hormones that help us to feel satiated after food. Understanding how the circadian rhythm affects health can be very effective to help your body operate its best.

The circadian rhythm is regulated by a part of the brain called the suprachiasmatic nucleus. This area uses approximately 20,000 neurons to influence hormonal activities in the body and brain. It is located near the pituitary gland in the hypothalamus, a region of the brain that is about the size of an almond. The suprachiasmatic nucleus receives signals from the eyes that tell it whether it is light or dark outside. This affects how the brain tells the body to operate. When the retina registers a lack of light, the production of melatonin increases to make you feel tired. This sleep hormone can affect many aspects of body function, including the microbe community in the gut.

Inside of our digestive system there live amoebae, fungi, viruses, and bacteria. This microbial community can involve over a thousand species and can have various impacts on health. The food we eat can alter the microbiome in our body, and so do the hormones we produce. These tiny microbes have their own circadian rhythm which functions very similarly to the one in our brain. Some play an active role during the day, while others are more active at night. They help to regulate our metabolism through affecting neurotransmitters, gut hormones, inflammatory responses, endotoxin levels, bile acids, branched chain amino acids (BCAAs), and short-chain fatty acids (SCFAs). These microbes have an important role in inflammatory and immune response, weight, and digestion. Through activity in our intestines, they come in contact with different cells that regulate biochemical processes like fatty acid production. The cells then send information to our circadian clock in our brain and other parts of our body which in turn affects our health.

The reverse can happen when we are introduced to stimuli that are not in keeping with our circadian rhythm. Disruptions to our circadian rhythm will also send signals to the gut which will disturb the gut microbes. This looped feedback can cause poor health. Our diet can also cause disruptions in the microbiome of our gut. A diet that contains high levels of Omega-3s and antioxidants and containing low levels of processed carbohydrates and inflammatory fats can help balance the circadian rhythms. However, a diet that is high in processed foods full of carbohydrates and unhealthy fats will cause a huge disruption in the gut bacterias' circadian rhythms. This can cause intestinal diseases such as gastroesophageal reflux disease (GERD), irritable bowel syndrome (IBS), or peptic ulcer disease. Circadian rhythm disruptions can also cause obesity, tumors, and accelerate aging. Avoiding these disruptions is very important to maintaining good health and preventing potentially harmful effects.

Eating a gut-friendly diet can help to keep these microbes from getting off track. This means including fermented foods into your diet. Kimchi, Sauerkraut, kombucha, and kefir will all help gut health by introducing healthy bacteria. Eating raw honey will help to get rid of bad bacteria, and a good probiotic supplement will improve gut health as well. This will all help feed the microbes and balance the presence of good bacteria and bad bacteria.

One of the best ways to regulate the microbial health of your gut is to incorporate time-restricted feeding. Time-restricted feeding involves consuming all of one's daily calories during a feeding window of 12 hours or less and fasting for the remaining 12 hours or more. The time restricted feeding method discussed most in this book is the 16:8 diet, but there are other variations such as the 12:12 and 14:10 methods. The 16:8 diet includes a 16-hour fasting window and an 8-hour feeding window. If you are fasting solely for gut health, and not for weight loss, a 12:12 or 14:10 schedule would be less restrictive. Although other health benefits of longer fasts, besides weight loss, should be taken into account as well. Usually, the fasting window during the time restricted feeding begins in the evening then lasts throughout the night and into the morning or afternoon when the fast is broken. Most people try to end their feeding window earlier in the late afternoon or early evening, but there are variations to this. For the purposes of regulating gut health, this method can be helpful in avoiding disruptions to the circadian rhythm by not eating during the nighttime hours. It can also be helpful because fasting allows the body to not be in a food processing state. This allows your gut microbes to take a break from digesting and absorbing food. Some doctors explain the relationship between fasting and gut health by comparing the body to a computer. Sometimes a computer gets slowed down due to corruptions, so we turn it off and allow it to reboot a few times. Give it a break and let it restart with everything in order. This is similar to how fasting helps our body. Sometimes we acquire issues that keep our body from operating at an optimal level, some minor issues and some major. By fasting, we give the system a break and allow it to sort out some issues while it reboots. This lets our "internal physician," as Hippocrates would say, do its work.

There are a few other ways to get your circadian rhythm back on track. In turn, it can help your gut health and prevent aging. The brain reacts to the environmental cues it receives, so to help it maintain its biological routine. We need to give it a more routine set of stimuli. A few things that will help your body clock even out are by scheduling your meals and exercise, being aware of light exposure, avoiding drugs or stimulants, and regulating your sleep schedule. Scheduling meals around the same times every day will help you digest your food better and help the circadian clock avoid confusion. If you follow a regular schedule, the brain will begin to predict when food is going to enter the body so it will send signals to the gut and liver, as well as the rest of the body, to get ready to process it. Eating during these times can optimize metabolic processes and allow for maximum food absorption. When your body is accustomed to performing a function at a specific time, stimulating that function at another time will yield less than optimal results, as well as confusing the part of the brain that controls it. By avoiding drastic variations in the times at which we eat, we process our food better and avoid impeding the routine of our circadian clock.

Scheduling exercise is also important because it can stimulate the body. Avoid exercising late at night when you are going to want the body winding down to sleep. Exercising in the morning can help wake you up for the day as well as taking advantage of the increase in fat burning and muscle building hormones that are present in the morning.

Being aware of light exposure is also very important for regulating your circadian rhythm. The suprachiasmatic nucleus in the brain receives light signals directly from the retina and uses them to determine how to stimulate hormone production. Light represses the production of melatonin, the sleep hormone, which can make it harder to sleep if you are surrounded by light at bedtime. Closing the blinds after dark to block out street lights and dimming household lights at night can help the body know it's nearing time to sleep. Avoiding screen time on cell phones, tablets, televisions, and computers after dark are also important. This is not always possible, but at the very least allow one full hour away from screens before going to sleep. Many cell phones have a "night shift" mode that alters the coloring of the backlight to remove the "blue light" that is most harmful to the sleep cycle. There are also special glasses available, called "blue blockers," that can be worn to block out blue light in the hours before bed to allow for better sleep. In the morning, you can practice something called light therapy to tell your brain that "this is the start of the day and this is when your rhythm should start." This can be done by a doctor, or you can use over-the-counter light devices. This aids in allowing the brain to build a consistent rhythm.

It's also important to avoid drugs and stimulants that will change the sleeping and waking hours of the brain. While taking drugs is rarely advised, it is certainly not advised to consume stimulants late in the day or during hours when the circadian clock is telling the body to sleep. This list of "drugs" contains prescription stimulants, cocaine, and even caffeine. Nicotine is also considered a stimulant and should be avoided at night.

Adjusting your sleep schedule is one primary component in regulating your circadian clock. If you are someone who goes to sleep very late every night, moving your bedtime to earlier can greatly benefit your health and the quality of your sleep. However, if you normally go to sleep at 3 o'clock in the morning, it would be difficult to suddenly switch to lights out at 10:30 in the evening. It is recommended to adjust your sleep schedule slowly by scaling back your bedtime using increments of 15 minutes every second or third day. This will allow your body to adjust and make it easier to fall asleep at an earlier time.

When you are trying to sleep earlier, going to bed can seem like a chore. To avoid this, create a bedtime routine that relaxes you and makes you feel good about going to sleep. A warm bubble bath or a nice shower can relax your muscles, and soothing music or a podcast can relax your mind. Use products with relaxing scents like lavender and be sure you have bedding and pillows that are comfortable. The temperature in your room and the amount of light are also important. Try to make the room as dark as possible. Cover the flashing light of your alarm clock with some fabric or stick a piece of colored tape on the little green light of your phone charger. Ensure the room is not too warm, and use earplugs to block out noise if you are a light sleeper.

Going to sleep earlier will also help with waking up earlier. Having a consistent wake time that is incredibly beneficial to the brain's clock. Your clock does not know that it's Saturday and you are off work, it's just going about its normal schedule, so if you sleep in it will be confused at the change in routine.

The more reliable your sleeping and waking times are, the more regular your clock will be. This is why it's also important to avoid napping. I know, sometimes it can be tempting to take a quick power snooze when you are feeling that midday lull, especially if you are in the process of adjusting your sleep schedule to sleep earlier and wake up earlier. Sleeping during the day can confuse the circadian clock and make you less able to fall asleep when bedtime comes. Try exercise at times when you normally feel tired to stimulate yourself and help your body rest better when you sleep at night. Once you have a new and improved sleep schedule established, try not to stray from it. Keeping this routine consistent will keep the circadian rhythm from being thrown off. One disruption can cancel out all the progress you've been working for.

It may take some time to get your circadian rhythm completely in check, but if you do, you will see the benefits. This will improve your overall wellness and prevent metabolic disorders. Fasting has the profound effect of allowing your body to improve parts of its health without extraneous medicines. We discern that our bodies are sometimes more capable than we realize. Living in tune with our natural biological cycles gives our body the opportunity to do what it's designed to do, be healthy.

Chapter 5: Methods of Fasting

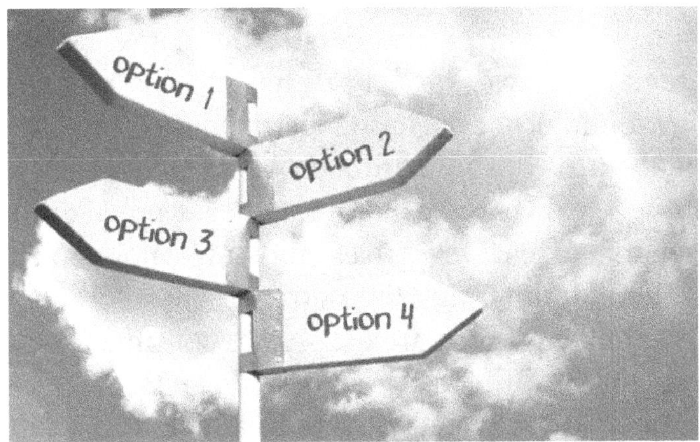

There are various methods of intermittent fasting, so there is bound to be a method that suits your lifestyle. Some methods are more intense than others, and it is to be noted that the fasts that yield more radical results are generally the fasts that require more radical dedication. However, even small fasts can boost your metabolism and help you see results. Some methods, like the 5:2 diet, do not require a full fast, but rather a large decrease in the number of calories consumed on fast days. The 16:8 diet simply involves skipping one meal a day. These two methods are generally considered the least daunting and are good ways to introduce your body to fasting. Other methods include the "eat - stop – eat" diet (which involves a 24-hour fast once or twice each week), alternate day fasting, and the warrior diet. Which method you choose depends on various factors like your schedule, special events, responsibilities to feed others, biology, weight loss or muscle gain goals, and workout routine. Whatever needs you have to meet, there is a method of intermittent fasting that can suit your life.

5:2 Diet

If completely depriving your body of calories seems too scary, give the 5:2 diet a try. The premise is simple, eat normally for five days out of the week and drastically reduce calorie intake on the remaining two days. For men, it is recommended to consume around 600 calories on fasting days. For women, it is recommended to consume around 500 calories. You can meet this calorie goal with whatever foods you like, but it's recommended to eat vegetables and low-calorie proteins to ensure you are still getting the nutrients your body needs. On the five feeding days, you are allowed to continue on a normal diet. If you are wanting to see quicker results, it's not best to overeat during these five days or to eat foods that will not fuel your body well. Not only can this prevent your body from reaching the caloric deficit you are aiming for, but it also means that on the fasting days, but your body also will not react as well to the reduction in energy. It's also ideal to make sure the fasting days are not consecutive. Eating for five days, then only allowing yourself a total of 1000-1200 calories in the remaining 48 hours can leave the body feeling weak. Separate the two fasting days by making sure there is at least one, if not more, feed day between them. When you are new to fasting, it's not encouraged to jump right in with both feet. Test the waters first by implementing a 5:2 diet. Begin by incorporating one calorie restricted day per week, then work your way up to incorporating two days. If you want to give the 5:2 diet a try but do not know how to get started, worry not. This book contains a 14 day 5:2 diet meal plan that you can follow to begin implementing a 5:2 eating schedule.

Every diet has a few downsides, and some people will struggle more than others. The fact that the 5:2 diet does not require a full fast from calories can actually make it a bit harder to get used to. Meeting a small calorie count rather than avoiding food altogether can leave one feeling hungrier and more focused on the lack of food. Fasting from food in its entirety affects the production of hunger hormones, and over time your body will start to get less hungry during your fasting periods. When you are restricting calories dramatically but still eating, this change in hormones does not occur. You may be left feeling the effects of your hunger much more than someone who chooses another fasting routine. During other methods of fasting, it can also help to distract yourself from the food you are not eating. The 5:2 diet does not allow this quite as much. In fact, if you are serious about your weight loss goals and desire to make the most of your minuscule calorie allotment for the day, you may find that you are even more focused on food than normal. It's also important to note that your fast days should be scheduled on days when you won't be over-exerting yourself. Because you are giving yourself less fuel, intense workouts or high levels of physical exertion will be difficult on the body. Yoga and light exercise like walking may be ideal for the two days during which your calorie count is low.

16:8 Diet

The 16:8 diet is another method that may allow you to introduce intermittent fasting into your diet without being overwhelmed. The 16 stands for the sixteen-hour "fast" period, and the 8 stands for the eight-hour "fed" period. The 16:8 method basically involves sacrificing one meal a day, and it's up to you whether that meal is in the morning or evening. When you finish eating for the day, you simply wait 16 hours before beginning to eat the next day. If you sleep a standard eight hours a night that already takes care of half of your sixteen-hour fast period! Let's say you wake up in the morning and have a cup of coffee or tea to start your day. Try to avoid adding sugar or milk, but it's widely accepted that if you consume less than 50 calories during the fasting period, your body will continue to benefit from fasting without entering a fed state. So, you can have your morning beverage, and good on you if you can keep your tea or coffee plain. Then around 1 o'clock p.m., you can eat lunch. You can snack if you want in the afternoon, then eat an evening meal. Because you started eating at 1 o'clock, you should finish eating by 9 o'clock that evening. During this eight-hour fed period, you can consume a full day's worth of calories. It's important to ensure that you are staying hydrated between 9 o'clock and 1 o'clock the following afternoon. Water intake should be increased slightly beyond the normal level to compensate for the fluids that would normally be absorbed by food consumption. Flip this schedule if you are a person who really needs to eat in the morning to be fueled for your day. You can break your fast at 8 a.m. and begin fasting again at 4 p.m. This can allow a breakfast, some snacks, and a late lunch, or even a small lunch and an early dinner before you begin fasting again.

Allowing sixteen hours without feeding your body will give it an opportunity to use the calories in the food it has consumed as well as burning stored fat for fuel. You can modify the 16:8 diet to fit into your schedule and meet your personal needs. Many people find this diet to be the least restrictive form of intermittent fasting because it does not require any alteration in the number of calories consumed and a standard meal schedule is able to fit well into an 8-hour block.

Other Time Restricted Eating Diets

If you are a beginner wishing to implement this method, you can start by incorporating a larger eating window and gradually shortening it over time. The 16:8 method is part of a group of fasting schedules referred to as "time-restricted eating" which also includes the 12:12 method and 14:10 method. The 12:12 method is very similar to a schedule many people already follow and may be a good start if you've never tried time-restricted eating before. Start with a 12-hour eating window, then after a week, you can take away 2 hours. Now you are practicing the 14:10 method. After another week, give 16:8 a try. Some people even choose to go further with their time restrictions and incorporate an 18:6 or 20:4 schedule.

It is up to you to choose how far you would like to take your schedule restrictions. The most important thing to take into account when considering your options is the health of your body. Take your time in adjusting to fasting to avoid unnecessary stress on the body and always be sure your body is healthy enough for fasting before implementing any changes.

It is important to note that if you wish to incorporate physically demanding exercise into your day, you should be aware of how your body reacts to working out in a fasted state versus a fed state and schedule your meals and workouts accordingly. Some people choose to do fasted workouts for a variety of reasons, and some find that their bodies are simply not adequately fueled for such workouts during the fasting period. Your fasting method should be adapted to suit your life, so pay attention to your body and take it into consideration. Pushing your body to work out when you have less energy due to fasting can lead to ineffective workouts and even injury. Many sports nutritionists advise choosing a fasting schedule that coincides with your ideal workout schedule so you can fuel your body immediately before or after exercise. If you are practicing the 16:8 method by skipping breakfast, this may mean working out in the afternoon or evening. Many people prefer to work out in the morning when human growth hormone levels are naturally highest. If this is the case for you, you may choose to implement your feeding window in the morning and begin your fast in the afternoon rather than the evening.

Alternate Fasting

Alternate day fasting, or the "every other day diet," is fairly self-explanatory. Eat for one full day, fast for one full day, repeat. This does not mean to fast from the moment you wake up until the end of the day but eat three square meals the next day. When practicing alternate day fasting, you should eat at least one meal every day. This may mean eating breakfast before 9 o'clock in the morning then abstaining from food until the same time the next day, or it could involve eating dinner by 7 o'clock in the evening and abstaining until 7 o'clock the following evening. Whatever time works best for you can be the beginning or ending time of your 24-hour fasting and feeding windows. This diet drastically reduces the calorie intake over the whole week because you are removing multiple days' worth of calories from the equation. Fasting for a full day between feast days allows the body to spend more time in a fat burning unfed state. On feasting days, you can eat whatever you'd like. For optimal weight loss, sticking to a healthy diet and not bingeing with carbs or unhealthy snacks is ideal. Some people practice this method with the same caloric restrictions as the 5:2 diet, so on fasting days, they are allowed 500 to 600 calories. Some studies have shown that this level of calorie intake is easier to maintain than full fasts and overall it is similar in effectiveness.

The "every other day" method has not proven to be any more effective than utilizing a diet that involves daily calorie restriction, but some people find it easier to restrict every other day so they can still enjoy an unrestricted diet half of the time. Both will yield similar fat loss results, but the intermittent fasting method has shown more successful in preserving muscle mass. This muscle mass is crucial to the burning of calories. It has also been shown that, in some cases, following this method can cause the body to feel less hungry during restricted periods than it would on a standard, calorie restrictive diet and can decrease the likelihood of binge eating on feast days. Hormones such as ghrelin that cause the body to feel hungry when it is fasting can decrease, and the hormones that cause it to feel satiated increases. The concern with this diet is that intermittent fasting is not always a permanent lifestyle choice and a diet like this can increase the likelihood of bingeing later on. When you are used to a full binge one day and a full restriction the next, you can lose touch with what true hunger or satiety feels like. When you resume consuming food on a daily basis, the eating habits you may have become accustomed to bingeing and may lead to weight gain.

This method is also not ideal for women. The female body reacts differently than the male body to extended periods of fasting. A full 24 hours of fasting is riskier for women, but still within the allowed time frame. Extended fasts in women can change hormone levels drastically and over time can cause permanent damage to the reproductive system, possibly even leading to infertility. If you are a woman who would like to utilize this type of eating schedule, it is possible, but it's important to understand the risks associated with it. It is also important to avoid implementing such a long period of food avoidance if your body is not already accustomed to fasting. Start by fasting for 12 hours, then gradually increase the fasting window until you reach 24 hours to avoid a major shock to the body that can cause hormonal imbalances with potentially dangerous side effects.

Eat-Stop-Eat Diet

If you do not want to fast quite as consistently, try incorporating a 24-hour fast into your diet once or twice a week. This method is called the "eat - stop - eat" diet. The 24 hour fasting period should be scheduled so that you are consuming some form of sustenance every day. For instance, let's say you eat breakfast at 8:30 in the morning on Tuesday morning. You finish eating by 9 o'clock and begin your fast. At 9 o'clock in the morning on Wednesday morning, you can break your fast. Incorporating this type of fasting into your lifestyle once or twice a week can allow the same type of caloric deficit as other methods while not interfering as much with normal day-to-day activities. This method may be ideal if you like to do heavy workouts on many days of the week. Incorporating fasting on your rest days can allow you to fuel yourself well on work days and decrease consumption on days when you are burning fewer calories. In the same form as other methods, sticking to healthier foods on feast days can help to achieve the results while also avoiding feelings of weakness and lethargy during the fasting period.

The eat - stop - eat method will be helpful in reaching a caloric deficit and losing weight. However, this method may not yield the same caliber of results as others because the fasting is less consistent. The body will remain more accustomed to being in a fed state and therefore not gain quite the same level of benefits as more frequent fasting. It is still an effective method and will still be beneficial to the body's processes. Eat - stop - eat may be a good option for you if you are new to fasting or if you find it difficult to add a fasting schedule into your busy life.

Some people extend their fast little by little until it lasts for a duration of multiple days to increase the amount of time the body is in a fat burning state. Long-term fasting has been shown to dramatically increase levels of the human growth hormone and noradrenaline. These two hormones are essential to fat burning, muscle growth, muscle preservation, energy levels, mental clarity, cellular repair, and anti-aging. Extended fasting also allows the body to enter and remain in a state of ketosis which will burn more stored fat and increase the rapidity of weight loss. It is wise to consult a doctor before incorporating long fasting periods into your lifestyle. For women, fasting for more than 24 hours at a time can have adverse effects on hormone levels and may cause permanent damage to the body. It may also not be smart if you have health problems that affect your blood sugar levels, such as diabetes. This can increase the risk of diabetic ketoacidosis and other potentially harmful illnesses associated with drastic changes in blood glucose levels. When you break your fast, the drastic change in blood sugar can be dangerous. Being aware of what is happening inside of your body is key to approaching fasting healthily. Long-term fasting can be beneficial, but it should not be attempted if your body is not healthy enough for it.

Warrior Diet

One of the more extreme methods of intermittent fasting is the Warrior Diet. The Warrior Diet is based on a theory that humans are biologically built to consume and process food in line with their circadian clock. The diet consists of eating one calorically dense meal every evening and fasting for the rest of the day. This is based around the belief that "warriors" of antiquity spent their time fighting, hunting and generally taking care of business throughout the majority of the day, so they ate much less during that time. Therefore, they would end their days indulging in a larger meal. In this same way, individuals who practice the Warrior Diet fast for the majority of every day. Generally, this follows a 20:4 method, with a twenty-hour fasting window and a four-hour feasting window. During the 4 hours, individuals consume a high number of calories. This can lead some people to choose unhealthy foods, but it is recommended to eat a healthy, balanced meal, especially if you will be exercising during your fasting period. Fueling your body properly will help you get optimal results and stay as healthy as possible while practicing intermittent fasting. During the 20-hour fast period, you do not have to avoid food entirely. Small snacks made up of raw vegetables or fruits, boiled eggs, and dairy products are encouraged, and you can drink as many calorie-free beverages as your warrior's heart desires. This includes tea, coffee, diet sodas, and of course lots and lots of water.

The Warrior Diet was created by an ex-member of the Israeli Special Forces who found inspiration in his time as a soldier and carried his knowledge and experience into the field of fitness and nutrition. However, the creator of this diet admits that it is not based on science and the amount of research around it is nearly non-existent. This does not necessarily mean that it isn't effective, but it is a good point to remember when considering this method.

Many people who practice the Warrior Diet incorporate exercise into their routine during the fasting period. This can be an effective way to build muscle, but it carries potentially harmful side effects. Pushing the body to its limits when it is low on fuel (food) can cause fatigue and dehydration, as well as decreasing your overall ability to perform which may lead to injury. This can also lead to a condition called hypoglycemia which is essentially dangerously low blood sugar. Hypoglycemia can lead to problems of varying severities ranging from confusion, increased clumsiness, trouble forming words, and dizziness to seizures and possible death. If you have type 1 diabetes or are on medication designed to lower your blood sugar, you should never attempt this diet. Again, it is important to consult your doctor before trying to incorporate a fasting regime into your lifestyle. An extended fast such as this also increases the likelihood of binge eating and consuming foods that are not rich in the nutrients necessary to fuel the body. When you are consuming a full day's worth of calories in 4 hours, opting for a carb-heavy meal full of processed food may seem appealing. Ensuring that your body is receiving the proper vitamins and minerals to maintain its functions is crucial to a healthy practice of intermittent fasting. Incorporating a meal prep plan into your Warrior Diet can help to avoid this issue and increase your likelihood of success.

Practicing any method of intermittent fasting is not recommended for people who may suffer from eating disorders. Any restrictive diet is not suggested for people with a tendency to over-restrict calories. Also, most people do not use intermittent fasting as a lifelong commitment, so someday they will probably stop practicing it. After you become accustomed to fasting, eating on a normal schedule can cause unwanted weight gain. You may lose touch with your ability to sense when you are truly hungry or full, and you may become accustomed to eating higher calorie meals. If you are not careful, this may lead to overeating which can bring about feelings of shame or regret that can negatively affect mental health. In individuals who are at risk of disordered eating, the negative emotions connected to this can lead to bingeing and purging behaviors.

Depending on the state of your health, your lifestyle, your weight loss or muscle gain goals, and your reaction to fasting, there is likely a method of intermittent fasting that suits your needs. The 5:2 diet and time restricted eating methods like the 16:8 are ideal for beginners and have much fewer risks attached. If you want fast, drastic results, the Warrior Diet may be ideal for you. All of these methods will help you lose fat. Some will help you lose more fat, more quickly, and some will help you build and maintain muscle mass more effectively. You do not have to stick to one method forever. The beauty of fasting is that it can be done in whatever way suits your lifestyle the best and can be catered individually to your wants and desires.

Chapter 6: Fasting to Lose Weight

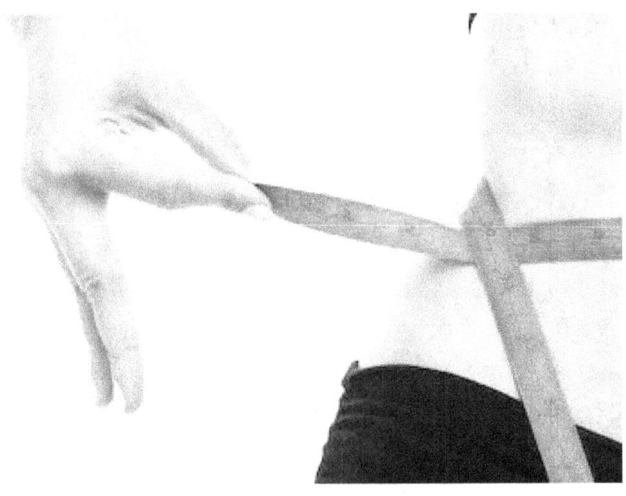

Any form of intermittent fasting will help you lose weight. The reason behind this is simple: to lose weight, you need to achieve a caloric deficit, and if you are not eating, you are decreasing the number of calories consumed. This makes fasting a great tool for weight loss, but there are other ways to enhance the effects of fasting and achieve the results you are looking for. Adding exercise to your intermittent fasting lifestyle will help you lose weight faster. Burning some calories that have been taken in will lead to a higher caloric deficit, and also increase levels of sweat that causes a loss in water weight.

If you maintain a healthy caloric intake during feeding hours, avoiding food during fasted hours will help you reach a caloric deficit. This means that you are consuming fewer calories than your body is using. To make up the difference, your body will use the energy in stored fat to fuel the processes it needs to sustain. Binge eating carb heavy, calorie dense, and unhealthy foods during fed hours can lessen this deficit, so for optimal weight loss, it is suggested that you also ensure that you are incorporating healthy meals into the equation. Decreasing the number of carbs you eat will avoid adding new fat stores. You'll be burning fat and also avoiding making more. Keeping insulin levels low will also help you burn more fat.

Food Choices

Fasting naturally lowers insulin levels and increases insulin sensitivity so your body will be absorbing sugars effectively. If you are consuming foods that cause insulin spikes, the body can start to store more fat rather than burning it. Wholesome, unprocessed foods are the most effective for avoiding this issue. When you go to the grocery store, the whole foods are generally located in aisles on the outside perimeter of the store. This is where you'll find fresh fruits, vegetables, and proteins. There are, of course, foods located on the inner aisles that can also benefit your diet, but the majority of a diet that will burn fat contains these whole foods. Knowing how macronutrients affect insulin levels will help you understand how to build your diet for optimal weight loss. Carbohydrates and dairy will have the largest impact on insulin because they are processed glucose. This means you'll want to avoid carbs as much as possible and lower your dairy intake. Proteins will have less of an impact on insulin levels. However, in the absence of sugars, the body will convert proteins into sugar using gluconeogenesis. Over consuming protein can cause insulin spikes as well, but less so than carbs. Fats have the least impact on insulin, so consuming more fats will fill you up without increasing insulin production. You can still incorporate dairy and carbohydrates into your diet without causing insulin spikes. Breaking your fast with a meal made of whole, unprocessed ingredients like vegetables will satiate your hunger so you can avoid overindulging in the more troublesome foods. Eat your vegetables and proteins first so that when you consume carbs and dairy, you will be doing so in smaller amounts.

The best way to be aware of what ingredients are going into your meals and ensure you are consistently consuming a healthy diet is to make the food yourself. This can be time-consuming. It can be difficult to work cooking into your schedule sometimes, especially if your eating window falls during the time of day where you are busy with work or other responsibilities. If this is an issue you come across, you may want to consider meal prepping. Meal prepping is the practice of taking a few hours on one or two of the less busy days of the week to prepare meals ahead of time. This does require a bit of an investment in both time and energy as it takes a large chunk out of the day, but the benefits it provides can help you to maintain a healthy diet, stick to your fasting schedule, and reach your weight loss goals.

The first step is to make a plan of what meals you want to consume in the coming days. It may help to make an inventory of the groceries you already have or to consider what foods you generally crave. It is also ideal to make meals that will refrigerate or freeze and reheat well as you won't be eating all the food right away. Once you've decided which meals you want to make, create a list of the ingredients you need. Choosing meals that contain common ingredients can cut down on the time and cost of meal prep. While shopping, remember the outer aisles of the grocery store are home to the more wholesome, single-ingredient foods. Note that when preparing multiple meals that contain chicken, try cooking all the chicken together. Once your meals are prepared, store them in the refrigerator or freezer and reheat when you are ready to eat! Another chapter of this book contains a more in-depth look at how to meal prep and how it will help you reach your goals.

There are two recommended fasting methods that may help you optimize your weight loss in a consistent, maintainable manner. The 5:2 diet is a great way to get started with intermittent fasting and is generally one of the less difficult methods to maintain over an extended period. The fact that an intake of calories is allowed even during the 2 fasting days may be helpful to your weight loss if you incorporate intense, fat burning exercise into your routine regularly. It's important to be aware of how you fuel your body, especially if it is being pushed to its limits. You can exercise during a fasting window that involves complete food avoidance and still be properly fueled, it just takes a little more planning ahead.

The other fasting method that may be ideal is a time restricted eating diet like the 16:8 method. This method involves fasting more consistently which increases the caloric deficit while also creating the benefit of a routine. It is, of course, not required that you follow a strict routine with any method, but the 16:8 diet allows the formulation of such. When trying to lose weight, building a routine can help you maintain the necessary consistency to achieve your ideal results. This does not just refer to the consistency in fasting, but also in eating healthy and exercising regularly. The more regularity you incorporate these aspects with, the more likely you will be to form healthy habits and achieve a maintainable healthy lifestyle that can positively benefit your weight loss and overall health. Other intermittent fasting methods will cause weight loss, and the results may be more rapidly visible, but these two types of eating schedules specifically can help you achieve healthy weight loss that is less likely to be undone if you stop practicing intermittent fasting.

Increasing the duration of your fasting window will also help you to burn more fat. After you become accustomed to fasting, carefully increase the duration of your fasting window. Fasting for 24 to 48 hours can increase the benefits of fasting exponentially. This should not be attempted in one drastic change. Gradually decrease the amount of time in your eating window by a couple of hours every week or two until you reach a point where you can fast for more than a full day. This will allow the levels of hunger hormones to decrease and enable you to fast longer without stressing your mind or your body too much. Extended fasting lowers insulin levels significantly and allows the body to burn more fat. A longer amount of time without consuming food will also increase the calorie deficit and allow for the use of more stored calories. Fewer meals eaten yields fewer calories added to the body. Some individuals think that decreasing the calorie consumption for a longer period will send the metabolism into preservation mode and decrease its effectiveness. This is based on the assumption that without adding calories to the body, the body will try to conserve the energy it has stored. Interestingly, the opposite happens. Noradrenaline production increases more with longer fasts. This can stimulate the metabolism by an increment of up to 14 percent. The body will use the stored glycogen it has and be able to metabolize calories more effectively when it is fed which will assist in weight loss. Noradrenaline also increases energy levels, alertness, and clarity in mental processes. This means that when you fast, you might expect to feel weak and depleted. Instead, your energy levels really aren't too terribly affected.

Exercise

Incorporating exercise into your routine will also help facilitate fat loss. Cardiovascular workouts are ideal for fat burning and will increase the calorie deficit. High-intensity interval training (HIIT) is an increasingly popular training style for fat loss that also stimulates the body's ability to metabolize glucose. HIIT workouts incorporate short intervals of high-intensity anaerobic exercise with short periods of rest in between. These type of workouts have been found to burn more calories than traditional endurance training. Even after the workout is finished, the body is still burning calories in a process called excess post-exercise oxygen consumption. Essentially, the body continues using up calories by working toward restoring itself to the same levels as prior to the workout. This leads HIIT workouts to be able to burn up to 15 percent more calories than other types of vigorous activities and becomes a useful tool in getting rid of body fat. In combination with intermittent fasting, high-intensity interval training is the best type of exercise to burn fat. Plus, you'll also improve cardiovascular health and endurance.

If you choose to include HIIT workouts into your routine while fasting, make sure you are not doing too much. High-intensity interval training isn't named this way it is for no reason. High-intensity workouts should not be done every day. Most trainers who recommend HIIT encourage alternating high-intensity workouts with low impact, steady-state exercises (LISS) such as walking or yoga. On these days you can also focus on stretching or foam rolling sore muscles. You should also be sure to incorporate at least one, if not more, rest days where the body can focus on recovery. Some people choose to exercise during fasted hours to make the most of the fat burning state the body has already entered. If you want to do this, listen to your body. HIIT is high intensity. The idea is to push your body to its limits for a short period, then rest and repeat. Pushing yourself when you are low on fuel can be dangerous. It can lead to sloppy, incorrect body form that increases the potential for injury. You may also feel weak, lightheaded, or dehydrated. Drink plenty of water, and if you know, you will be doing HIIT during your fast you should ensure that the last meal you consume before beginning your fast is full of the proper fuel. Eat a large number of vegetables, a moderate amount of protein, and plenty of healthy fats. Also be sure to incorporate some carbohydrates, but not too much. These carbs will replenish the glycogen stores in the muscles to be used during your workout.

Ketogenic Diet

Allowing the body to enter a state of ketosis will also improve the rapidity of weight loss. This is another benefit of a longer fasting window. Ketosis is a metabolic state in which the body uses fats for fuel rather than sugars. When you fast, your body uses the sugars that are stored in the liver and muscles as glycogen. After it has used all of this glycogen, the body still needs fuel, so it starts to use ketone bodies that the liver makes from breaking down fats. This way, the body begins to utilize stored fats for fuel and increases the weight loss. Fasting also lowers the levels of insulin in the blood because the body is not processing any sugar intake. Glycogen stores and insulin levels both affect the retention of water in the body. Each gram of glycogen that is stored in the muscles is accompanied by water in an amount ranging from 0.11 ounces to 0.14 ounces. High insulin levels cause the kidneys to retain water and sodium. By decreasing the levels of insulin in the blood, the kidneys receive the go-ahead to flush excess water. So, you'll lose water weight as well as using up fat stores.

One of the most effective ways to lose fat stores while fasting is to incorporate a ketogenic diet during your feeding window. A keto diet involves putting the body into ketosis and maintaining this metabolic state consistently to use up fat stores. In a normal diet, carbs are a main source for the glucose that fuels the body and feeds the cells. On a keto diet, the amount of carbohydrates that are consumed is drastically reduced. This causes it to look elsewhere for fuel which it finds in ketone bodies that are created by the liver when breaking down fats. Because of this metabolic change, the diet focuses heavily on consuming fats.

A standard keto diet incorporates a ratio of about 75 percent fats, 20 percent proteins, and only 5 percent carbs. There are a few variations of the ketogenic diet which include a cyclical diet, a targeted diet, and a high protein diet. A cyclical keto diet consists of only consuming keto approved macros for 5 days out of the week, but not following a keto diet on the remaining 2 days. A targeted keto diet consists of following a keto diet consistently but consuming the allotted carbs either directly before or directly after a workout. A high protein keto diet increases the amount of protein consumed during the day and decreases the amount of fat. If a standard ketogenic diet allows 75 percent fat and 20 percent protein, the high protein ketogenic diet will reduce the fat percentage to 60 percent and at the extra 15 percent to the protein intake to yield 35 percent protein. A cyclical ketogenic diet may be ideal for people following the 5:2 intermittent fasting diet as this may help you see better weight loss results.

A targeted ketogenic diet may be ideal for people who do strenuous exercise which depletes the glycogen stores in the muscles. This can allow the body to replenish the stores without coming out of a state of ketosis or turning muscle proteins into fuel. A high protein ketogenic diet may be ideal for people who which to build muscle. Building muscle can be difficult when in ketosis because the body needs protein to restore muscle fibers, but the lack of sugars require it to process protein to create glucose to fuel necessary processes. Increasing protein consumption can ensure that there is protein available for protein biosynthesis in the muscles.

When the body reaches a state of ketosis, it begins relying on fat for fuel rather than sugars. To maintain this state, feed the body just enough sugars to be utilized in cellular processes that cannot operate off of ketones and focus the majority of the diet on incorporating enough fats to fuel the body well. This process will allow the body to start using stored fats as fuel and increase the rapidity of weight loss. If you choose to include a focus on ketosis into your intermittent fasting lifestyle, you can purchase ketone testing kits to measure the levels of ketones in your blood, urine, or breath. This can help you to be aware of whether you are effectively maintaining a state of ketosis. On its own, the keto diet has been shown to have many of the same health benefits as fasting, including lowering insulin production and improving the lives of people living with type 2 diabetes. The diet was originally used in the treatment of children struggling with uncontrolled epileptic seizures. In some cases, these children are fasted to some degree for a couple of days before being put on a ketogenic diet to help the body enter ketosis faster. In the same way that research substantiating the health benefits of fasting is lacking at this point in time, the research surrounding health benefits of the ketogenic diet is not very abundant, but the studies that have been done show promise in many ways that coincide well with the effects of intermittent fasting, specifically in people with type 2 diabetes or problems with insulin resistance.

Fasting is known to increase the speed at which the body can reach a state of ketosis. By allowing the body to deplete the glycogen stores in your muscles, this uses the stored sugars and gets your body using ketones sooner. Many people choose to fast at least a few days before they start a Keto diet to establish the effects of the diet sooner. This also cuts down on the duration of the "Keto flu," a period of adjustment to the Keto diet in which one may be irritable and uncomfortable, as well as experiencing brain fog. Instead, many people begin to experience increased mental clarity when combining fasting and the Ketogenic diet.

Intermittent fasting is a very effective tool for weight loss. These tips will help you increase your weight loss more rapidly and see results sooner. Remember, while one major goal is to lose unwanted fat, the other major goal is to do so in a healthy and maintainable way so that the weight does not come back. Self-awareness regarding your body and your health is key to overall wellness. Listening to your body, fasting intermittently, fueling yourself properly, and exercising consistently is the formula for your desired weight loss. Every person's body is different, so find what works for your body and put it into action.

Chapter 7: Fasting to Gain Muscle

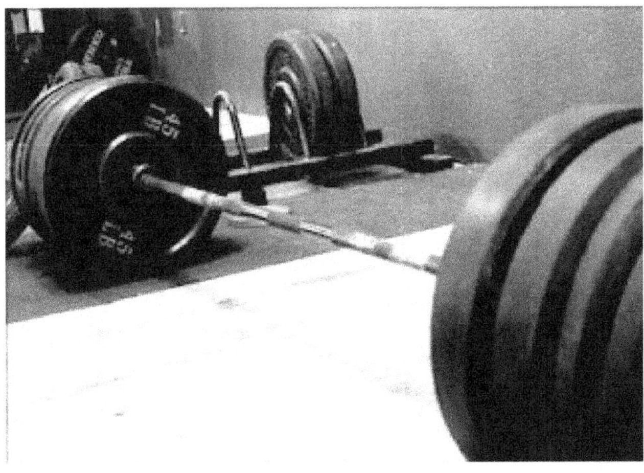

Intermittent fasting has shown to be just effective as a normal calorie restrictive diet in many ways. However, people who choose the intermittent fasting route have been shown to preserve muscle mass when losing fat while groups following a calorie-restricted diet for the same period lost both fat and muscle mass. There are a few ways to optimize muscle gain while on an intermittent fasting diet. It is very important to remember to consult a doctor before implementing any fasting regimens into your daily routine, especially when the goal results involve drastic weight loss or muscle growth. The most important key is to ensure that you are eating enough calories during your fed hours to compensate for calories lost during workouts.

The primary differences between trying to lose weight while fasting and trying to gain muscle while fasting are the way you exercise and the food you eat. Intermittent fasting is a beneficial tool when trying to gain muscle because you can lose fat and build muscle at the same time. The fasting is taking care of the fat loss, so you do not have to worry as much about burning fat in your diet and workouts. This changes the way you approach training. Your focus isn't on toning up to look better, it's on pushing your limits and getting stronger.

Lifting Weights

To build muscle, you need to lift heavy. If you are new to lifting, you can get stronger by lifting at least 60 percent of the maximum amount you can lift for one repetition. If you are doing bicep curls and 45 pounds is the maximum amount that you can successfully curl only once, then you need to be using at least 18 pounds for each set of reps to be building muscle. 60 percent of a single rep max is generally an amount that you can lift between 15 and 20 times in one set. This is not a particularly heavyweight, but as a beginner, it will help you build muscle.

As your body adjusts to lifting weights, consistently it becomes more difficult to build muscle. Over time, you will need to increase the percentage to at least 80 percent of your max to still be getting stronger and growing muscle. This is going to be an amount that you can't lift as many times. Rather than being able to do 15 to 20 reps in one set, you are not likely to be able to surpass 8 or 9 reps before you can't do anymore. So, the amount of weight you lift will affect muscle growth.

Another factor to take into account is the speed at which you lift this weight. Many people encourage slow, deliberate reps when trying to get stronger. This may be helpful in maintaining proper form, but it is not as effective in building functional strength or optimal muscle growth. Maintain controlled movements, but lift the weight faster and lower it slowly. Lifting faster yields more optimal muscle growth results because it uses more muscle fibers. This increases the amount of damage to the cells in the muscles which in turn increases the number of new, healthy cells that are added to repair them. So, lift heavier weights and lift them faster, but always maintain proper form.

If you reach a point in your sets where you cannot complete the reps without cheating on your form, stop. Reduce the weight if you'd like to finish out the set, but do not continue if you can't do it properly. Not using proper form can cause stress and injury to the muscles. When you are lifting heavy, you are working your strongest muscle fibers. When these stop doing their part, weaker muscle fibers start to bear a weight they are not cut out for. Damaging the muscles is part of building them, but injuring them is not a factor we want to add to the equation.

Feeding the Muscles

Muscles grow when you feed them. When trying to add muscle while fasting, you will need to increase the number of calories consumed during the fed hours. On days involving exercise, make sure the body is fed a surplus of calories so it can have the necessary fuel to perform protein biosynthesis. During training, muscle fibers are damaged. The body is always clearing out old, damaged cells and adding newer, healthier ones, so these damaged muscle cells get replaced with new ones. The body also has a nifty skill called adaptability. It wants to become better suited to dealing with whatever stimulus caused the damage to muscle fibers, so when the muscles fibers are repaired the body adds extra cells. This causes the muscles to get bigger. This is why bodybuilding athletes consume so much protein. The goal is to ensure that the body synthesizes more protein than is broken down. If more protein is destroyed than is being made, you will begin to lose muscle mass.

When you are fasting to lose weight, the larger the calorie deficit you achieve, the better the results. When you are fasting and trying to build muscle, you do not want a large calorie deficit. Instead, to gain muscle mass, you need to have a caloric surplus. This means that you'll need to increase the number of calories you eat during your feeding window, but that does not mean you should start stuffing your face with junk food to meet the necessary surplus.

Pay attention to the macronutrient levels in each meal to help you fuel your body in a manner that is helpful for your goals. Macronutrients include protein, fats, and carbohydrates. The ratio of macros that you incorporate into your meal plan can vary based on what diet you follow, but there are a few aspects that will be consistent across the board if you are trying to gain muscle. No matter what ratio of carbohydrates you incorporate into your diet, it is generally considered ideal to consume the majority of your carb allotment in your first meal after training. If you practice fasted training, ensure that your first meal after breaking your fast is the meal with the highest density of carbohydrates, contains plenty of protein and lower in fat. If you train during your feeding window, consume your carbs directly before working out for maximum muscle building benefit. Be sure to incorporate enough protein into your diet to fuel protein synthesis in the muscles to grow your lean mass. Eat multiple large, healthy and balanced meals throughout your feeding window to meet your macros and your calories.

What you eat is a huge part of any process where you are changing your body. It can sometimes be difficult to find the time to make enough food or eat frequently enough to maintain the calories you need to build muscle. Meal prepping large batches of food once or twice a week can ensure that you can spend more of your feeding hours eating to meet your macros and less time trying to prepare food. Find a day where you have an afternoon free and set aside that time to get your meals ready for the week. Think about what foods are dense in the macronutrients that you wish to consume so you can meet your goals easily and choose meals that will help you do so. Choose a few simple meals that you can make in bulk and eat repeatedly throughout the week to save time, money, and energy. Once you've chosen your meals, make a grocery list and ensure you have all the necessary ingredients. Then prepare a few days' worth of meals and store them in the freezer or refrigerator until you are ready to eat them. This will allow you to have food readily available when you want to feast. The next chapter will give you more information about how to meal prep and the benefits it adds to your intermittent fasting routine.

It is important to know how glycogen affects the muscles and how to ensure that the body does not begin using muscle mass for fuel through gluconeogenesis when fasting. It is highly unlikely that the body will reach this phase during shorter periods of fasting, but in prolonged fasts, it may happen. Keep this in mind when choosing a method of fasting. Gluconeogenesis is the process of turning things other than carbohydrates, i.e., protein, into sugars when sugars are lacking. This process won't occur until the stores of glycogen in the liver and muscles are depleted which can take up to 24 hours but can take as little as 6 hours when exercise is incorporated. After an intense workout with heavyweights, glycogen stores in the muscles are depleted. Glycogen is made from glucose, i.e., sugar. To replenish glycogen stores, the body needs glucose. This is when a targeted diet comes in handy. This method incorporates consumption of carbs after a workout to re-up the glycogen stores in the muscles. This ensures that muscles continue to grow well. At the very least, ensure that on days you are working out heavily you eat a larger number of calories and incorporate enough carbs to fuel the glycogen levels in the muscles.

Some trainers advise fasted training. Once your body is accustomed to fasting, it becomes better at nutrient partitioning. This means the body starts to send nutrients to the muscles where they are needed rather than sending them into storage in fat cells. Pushing muscles to their limits during the fasted state ensures that glycogen stores are depleted fully, which allows sugars to be processed into glycogen to replenish the muscles rather than stored. This can be beneficial to muscle growth. Just remember, muscles have to be fed to grow. Even if you continue fasting after you finish your workout, be sure that the first meal you eat when you break your fast after your workout is your largest meal of the day. However, do not immediately consume this huge meal the moment you break your fast. This can overwhelm the body and spike insulin levels. Break your fast with a small portion of food, wait approximately half an hour, and then consume the rest of your meal.

Incorporating fasting when trying to gain muscle is beneficial because it increases levels of human growth hormone (HGH) and noradrenaline as well as increasing insulin sensitivity. HGH increases the development of muscle mass and protects it from deterioration. Working out in the morning when HGH is released into the body will improve muscle gains and help you recover better from your workout. Athletes since the 1980s have been known to use extraneous doses of the human growth hormone to increase their muscle gains and muscle retention. High levels of HGH like these can have negative effects on the body, but the levels that show in the body during fasting are high enough to be beneficial, yet low enough not to be risky. Human growth hormone is essential to the cell renewal cycle and stimulates the growth of new cells which can help in the protein biosynthesis of muscles when damaged cells are replaced.

The increase in insulin sensitivity allows the body to process glucose more efficiently. This means that, in essence, your body will start sending the nutrients from your food directly to the muscles rather than storing them as fat. This will help the muscles grow and help decrease excess fat storage.

Noradrenaline is also increased as a biological response to needing to find food. When you fast, the body thinks that food must be scarce, so it increases this hormone that stimulates mental clarity and increases alertness and metabolism of stored energy. In theory, if you were a starving caveman who needed to find food, you would have a boost in energy so you can go out searching for it. The increase in noradrenaline coincides well with increased insulin sensitivity because noradrenaline stimulates the release of glucose from the glycogen stores in the liver and muscles. This allows the glucose in consumed food to be metabolized into glycogen to replenish these stores which means less glucose is stored in fat cells.

Best Fasting Method

The list of fasting methods that allow you to gain muscle is a little shorter than the list that helps you lose weight. When you are just trying to lose weight, any method will be effective even though some are more effective than others. When you are trying to build and maintain muscle mass, any method that involves a fast longer than 16 hours is out of the question. When you fast, the decrease in glucose intake causes your body to start using stored glycogen. Anywhere after 6 to 24 hours, the glycogen stores in your liver and muscles are depleted. If you are trying to gain muscle mass, it can generally be assumed that you do strenuous exercise that will deplete glycogen stores much faster. When those glycogen stores are depleted, the body starts to get its glucose from gluconeogenesis which makes sugar out of protein. This protein usually comes from damaged cells as well as connective tissues and skin which generally means that incorporating fasting shouldn't raise concerns about losing muscle mass. However, when you are trying to gain muscle mass, this process can prevent you from having sufficient protein to build up the muscle fibers. After 12 to 16 hours of fasting, gluconeogenesis becomes responsible for 100 percent of the glucose maintenance in the body. If you are maintaining a protein-rich diet during the fed hours, this may not be much of a concern for a short while. However, consistently allowing the body to break down proteins for sugars over hours upon hours can prevent growth in muscle mass and raise the risk of eventually losing the muscle mass that you have already developed.

Alternate day fasting, the eat - stop - eat diet, and the Warrior Diet all incorporate 24 hour fasting periods are not beneficial to gaining muscle mass. The extended fasting periods increase the amount of time the body is utilizing gluconeogenesis, as well as creating a larger calorie deficit for the week. The 5:2 diet is also not beneficial because it does not involve a time where food is avoided entirely. This decreases the hormonal benefits of fasting, such as the increase in human growth hormone which stimulates muscle growth and the metabolism. HGH is suppressed during eating, so consuming even the reduced number of calories allowed on 5:2 fast days will not allow the desired increases in this hormone. Also, when we want to build muscles, we need an excess of calories to do so. Drastically decreasing the number of calories consumed for 2 days out of the week will create a caloric deficit. This could be combated by increasing consumption on the other 5 days of the week, but overall this method is not recommended.

The most highly recommended intermittent fasting schedule for individuals who desire to reap the benefits of fasting while also gaining muscle mass is time restricted eating, primarily the 16:8 method. A fasting window of 12 to 16 hours will allow for the hormonal and fat burning benefits of fasting without being detrimental to muscle development. During the feasting hours, you should do just what the name says: FEAST. This does not mean to binge eat junk food, but you should eat often and eat largely. If you have trouble fitting enough food and calories into an 8-hour eating window, extend it by a couple of hours. Keep in mind that to build muscle you need a calorie surplus. If you'd like, you can fast following a 16:8 method for a few days out of the week and have an extended eating window on other days. The main goal is to ensure that for the week as a whole you have an average calorie intake that is greater than the number of calories lost. If you had a calorie deficit on some days, that's okay. Eat more on the other days to make up the difference.

Chapter 8: Meal Prepping for Intermittent Fasting

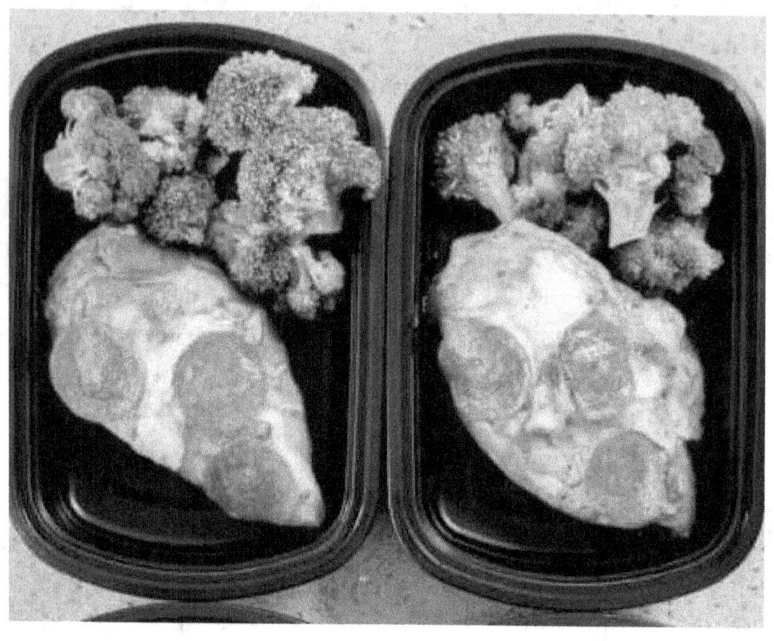

To get the optimal results from your fasting routine, you would want to incorporate exercise and a healthy diet into your lifestyle. To ensure that your body is properly fueled and your nutrient needs are met, it is best to pay attention to what you are consuming and whether or not you are meeting the calorie levels and macronutrients necessary for your desired effect. Planning meals ahead of time and preparing the foods you crave for will allow you to be more aware of your diet goals and achieve your ideal results. For example, the Keto diet will maximize weight loss, but it is not a requirement to follow any specific diet when you are practicing intermittent fasting. If you do not binge eating junk food on your feast days, you are likely not going to undo the effects of your fast days.

By adding meal prepping to your schedule, the stress of figuring out how to meet your calories and macros each day goes out the window. Spend one Sunday afternoon grocery shopping and preparing pre-portioned meals for the week, put them in the freezer or refrigerator, and eat when you need them. It's simple, saves time and money, and helps you make better diet choices throughout the week. Plus, with consistent practice of almost any fasting method, you'll decrease the number of meals you need to prepare by nearly a third, if not more. If you lead a busy life, and meal prepping can make incorporating intermittent fasting into that schedule much easier. And the best thing, you do not need to be super strict about how you do it. Putting excess stress on yourself about counting calories or macros can be discouraging and leave you uninspired to meal prep or to stick to a diet and eating schedule. Preparing a few pre-portioned meals for breaking your fast on your workday lunch breaks may be enough meal prep for you. This chapter will provide a resource to understand how meal prepping works, and how you can incorporate it into your lifestyle in the way that works best for you. It will also provide a guide on how to properly store and reheat different types of foods so you can enjoy your food as much as possible.

Meal Prep Considerations

Choosing foods that fuel the body well during your fed hours can help to decrease weakness and fogginess during fasted hours. If you plan to have an intense workout in the morning, replenish your glycogen stores with a dose of carbohydrates during your last meal the night before, or eat your most carb heavy meal of the day immediately after breaking your fast. Carbs before a workout will allow the body to produce glycogen that can be used during the workout, and carbs afterward can replenish glycogen stores. On the other hand, during other fed hours, eating a diet that is high in fat and lower in carbohydrates will prevent insulin spikes and allow the body to use the sugars it has in storage which will stimulate proper nutrient metabolism. Plan your meals around these concepts to ensure that you are making the most out of your meals.

If you incorporate a method like the 5:2 diet that allows consumption of a certain number of calories throughout the day, it can help to plan those calories ahead of time to ensure you are making the most of your allotted amount. 500 calories of junk food and 500 calories of protein and vegetables will have evidently contrasting effects on how your body functions during your fast. Make sure to eat vegetables or fruits that are naturally low in calories, as well as incorporating low-calorie sources of protein. Preparing small, low-calorie, nutrient dense foods in pre-portioned containers will help you feed your body what it needs and make fasting days more bearable. It may also help to schedule your intake to spread the calories out over the whole day and optimize your meals.

Meal prepping takes an investment of both time and energy, but the benefits outweigh the cost. Dedicate a free afternoon to prepare meals that will easily store in the refrigerator or freezer, and you won't have to worry about preparing them throughout the week. When you are hungry, reheat the food and enjoy a home-cooked meal without the hassle. Preparing so many meals ahead of time may be a daunting idea, but it's truly a simple process. First, decide what meals you plan to eat throughout the week. Then, create a grocery list for the meals and get all the ingredients. Make all of your meals, store them, and enjoy later. Creating a meal plan will take out a lot of the guesswork.

What foods you choose to prepare can vary heavily based on what results you are trying to achieve. If you are trying to lose weight, choose meals and snacks that are lower in calories to increase your caloric deficit. Decrease the number of carbohydrates to avoid insulin spikes. For those who are trying to build muscle, choose foods that are higher in calories so you can meet your surplus, and make sure to incorporate carbs to fuel your workouts and protein to feed your muscles.

Create a meal plan that includes only a few variations of meals for the week to decrease the complexity of your meal prep. Using similar ingredients in different recipes can cut shopping costs and preparation times. For instance, if you have two meals that involve chicken you can buy the chicken in bulk and cook it together. Once you have decided on which foods you'd like to prepare, create a list of what items you need to get and in what quantities. Then, take note of what ingredients you already have. Check those off of the list, then do the grocery shopping to get the rest. For the healthiest diet, remember that these are natural, unprocessed whole foods. Most of your ingredients should be these foods. When you have all of your ingredients, prepare your meals and store them for later use.

While you are cooking, you may find it helpful to try multitasking. If you want to make two recipes in the oven that need to be baked at the same temperature, try cooking both at the same time if your oven has space for 2 pans. Be sure to pay attention to the required cooking time for each recipe, especially if they will be done at different times. Using a kitchen timer or cell phone timer can be helpful. If you are concerned about being able to safely bake two meals at once, do not worry. That is not the only way to multitask. If one recipe calls for a longer cooking or simmering time, choose a recipe that can be made in the meantime. The goal of meal prepping is to save time, avoid stress, and keep you on track to your results. Using your time efficiently will help things go smoothly and avoid any discouragement or frustration.

Pre-Portioning

Individual portioning is a frequently practiced method of preparing meals in advance. With this method, food is prepared and portioned out into containers that hold one serving worth of each food. These containers are refrigerated or frozen until you need them. Pre-portioning meals is a good choice for individuals who are trying to lose the optimal amount of weight during their fasting. When you want to reach a caloric deficit, preparing a container of food that contains the proper number of servings for one meal can help you have an easier time keeping track of the calorie content. This can help to cut out the guesswork of trying to figure out the calories per serving later on.

You can use any type of food storage container that you'd like, but when freezers and microwaves are involved, you want to be sure your container of choice can withstand both. You'll want a dish with an airtight lid, and partitions that allow you to separate different foods can be an added bonus.

Depending on what method of intermittent fasting you practice, you may not need to make as many meals for the week, but when each meal has its own separate container, it may be difficult to find space to store even a smaller than an average number of meals. You do not have to pre-portion every meal, but it is a very helpful tool for days when you are busy at work or will be on the go.

A make-ahead meal like casserole or soup might be a good option if you do not have the space to store individual servings. With this method, a full meal is cooked, but it isn't separated into individual portions. If you are preparing meals for the whole family, this can be an ideal way to save time. A pot of soup can be frozen for up to 3 months. You can store the whole pot as one, but once you defrost it, you may not want to refreeze it. Divide it into containers that hold a week's worth of servings, then you can defrost one container for the week and store it in the fridge until it's consumed. This can be good for low-calorie diets as many soups are lower in calories. Casseroles and pasta can be prepared in the same way.

Another meal prep hack is to cook large batches of foods that are eaten frequently. If you are trying to build muscle and you know that you are particularly fond of one specific protein-rich chili recipe, triple the recipe and store the excess in glass jars in your freezer. This can keep for months and can help you keep your diet on track should you come across a week where you do not have time to meal prep. You already have a store of some of your favorites in the freezer. This can also help in saving money. If you are making a large quantity of something, you can buy ingredients in bulk. This can generally decrease the price per unit of each ingredient.

Cooking all of your meals ahead of time can save you hours in the long run, but that's not ideal for everyone. It can still be beneficial to incorporate meal prep techniques even if you do not want to precook a week's worth of meals. Precook proteins like turkey breast or chicken, but not meats like shrimp which do not reheat well. If there are ingredients that you frequently use in cooking, you can prepare them ahead of time to make meal assembly easier. If you like to top your salad with sliced almonds or walnut pieces, take a time out of your afternoon to cut up enough nuts for a week or two. You can also pre-dice onion or garlic for savory dishes, or slice up vegetables, so they're ready to roast. If you are following the 5:2 meal plan at the end of this book and you want to have a ginger, apple and carrot smoothie for breakfast on one of your restricted days, prepare for this by placing the portioned ingredients into a plastic resealable bag and putting them in the freezer. When you are ready to make a smoothie, you can take the baggie out of the freezer and dump the contents into a blender with some water.

Meal prep is generally a very simple process to understand. In fact, simplicity is one of the key ingredients to enjoying the benefits of meal prep in your intermittent fasting lifestyle. You do not have to only use one method of meal prep, and it's not a strict science. Planning makes reaching your goals much easier. Plan which foods you'd want to cook, make a list of the groceries you will need to get before you can make them, plan ways to multitask and finish your preparations efficiently, and plan the space you will use to store the food. Do not try to incorporate a different gourmet recipe for every meal of the week, and also do not choose meals that you know will not be appealing more than once. Find a balance that works for you.

It is very helpful to have food prepared in advance, but sometimes it can be less than ideal to eat a reheated meal. You do not want every food you eat to feel like you are eating leftovers, so it's important to learn how to properly store your foods and reheat them for the ideal level of tastiness. If you are avoiding food for hours on end, why not make sure that eating is an enjoyable experience when you do allow yourself to do it.

Proper Storage

You'll want to leave a little room in the top of the container full of food before freezing, but not too much. A plastic food storage container may suffice, and these can usually be purchased in bulk either online or at some supermarkets. Glass food storage containers are usually preferable because they tend to seal tighter, easier to clean, and less likely to stain. Plastic Ziploc bags will also come in handy for some foods, as well as plastic food wrap and aluminum foil.

If you want to freeze your food, be sure your freezer is colder than 0 degrees Fahrenheit (-17.8 degrees Celsius). For refrigerated foods, be sure the refrigerator is colder than 35 degrees Fahrenheit (1.7 degrees Celsius). Frozen meals can keep for months at a time, depending on ingredients. Refrigerated meals generally need to be consumed within the first 24 hours to 3 days.

Safe Thawing and Reheating Methods

Once you know how to store food to maintain freshness, you'll need to learn how to thaw and reheat each meal most effectively. Reheating methods include microwaving, stove top heating, and baking in the oven. If your meals are already cooked before being stored, reheating can change the texture of certain foods, and if not done properly it can become unappetizing. Sometimes this knowledge will change the way you prepare a meal. If a food is being prepared to be frozen for later consumption, leaving certain ingredients undercooked or excluded can allow for optimal reheating.

If you are using uncooked ingredients, it is important to thaw them properly before cooking to ensure thorough cooking and avoid contamination. The healthiest way to thaw any frozen food is to place the frozen goods in the refrigerator overnight before the day you wish to use them. This method allows the food's temperature to rise slowly and ensures the food thaws evenly. If you place frozen food on the counter at room temperature to thaw, the food can begin to breed bacteria as it reaches the temperature of its surroundings. If you are on the go, take a pre-portioned meal out of the freezer in the morning before work can allow it to thaw enough by lunchtime that it can be reheated easily. The food shouldn't reach a concerning temperature during such a short time, but you should ensure the food is heated to a proper temperature before being eaten, just in case.

Meats

Meats store very well in the freezer and maintain their integrity when reheated. If they are stored properly, both uncooked and cooked meat products can be kept in the freezer for up to 3 months without losing their quality. Patties made out of ground meats, like hamburgers or sausages, should be laid flat on parchment paper and frozen until solid. Then you can take the patties and stack them in an airtight container or wrap them in foil to store. This can be done with uncooked or cooked meats. Before cooking or consuming meats that have been frozen, they should be allowed to thaw thoroughly.

It's ideal to thaw meat in the refrigerator overnight before heating. If you forget to do this or do not have time, put the meat in an airtight plastic bag and let it sit under a stream of cold water until it's thawed. Do not use warm or hot water because this can raise the temperature of parts of the meat too drastically and lead to the breeding of bacteria. The better thawed your meat is before you reheat it, the faster it will reach the desired temperature.

Meat can dry out easily in the microwave or oven, so shorter cooking time during reheating is better. If you want to use a microwave to warm your meal, cut the meat into smaller pieces, so it heats faster. Also, put a slightly dampened paper towel over the plate to add a little moisture.

Stovetop reheating might be a bit more ideal. Foods like steak or chicken breast do not microwave well. Adding a small portion of butter to the pan with the mean can keep it moist, or you can use water if you'd like to avoid the extra fats. This tip also translates to reheating in the oven. Add butter to the pan with the food and reheat it on a low temperature until it's ready. This is the best option for warming meat. It might take a bit longer than a microwave or stovetop, but it will be more likely to maintain the flavor and texture of your meat. For meat, the oven is the most ideal warming method, followed by the stovetop and then the microwave.

Vegetables

Meat and veggies are two major components of a healthy diet. Cooked vegetables may have an odd texture after being frozen. If you know that you will be freezing vegetables for later consumption, do not cook them completely when you are preparing them. Leave them slightly underdone to prevent sogginess when reheating. If you are using a microwave to warm them up, put a small amount of water or a damp paper towel on or near the plate before warming. This will create steam that will heat the vegetables.

Using a stovetop rather than a microwave is slightly more ideal. Put the vegetables in a pan with a tiny amount of olive or coconut oil and stir them while they cook. This will yield crispier vegetables. In the case of veggies, the oven is not the best option, but it can still be used. Drizzle a bit of oil on the vegetables and warm them on a low heat. This will also yield crispier vegetables. For vegetables, the stovetop is the most ideal warming method, followed by the oven and then the microwave.

Casseroles

Casseroles that are prepared in advance for freezing and reheating can also be left slightly undercooked and will finish cooking during the reheating process. They can be frozen for up to 3 months. Make sure that these dishes are thoroughly thawed before you warm them. Heating frozen casserole without thawing will leave a lot of excess water. Casseroles with a high vegetable content may have extra water after thawing, so drain this before warming the food. It is also important to always heat food to a high temperature, which may involve cooking the food a bit longer and allowing it to cool before eating. Use a single portion rather than heating the entire casserole, simply cut one portion from the frozen food and place it in a container in the refrigerator to thaw.

To reheat casseroles in a microwave, you'll need to separate it into portions and microwave them for a couple of minutes on high. Microwaving is more likely to leave this dish slightly watery, even if it's thawed beforehand.

Warming casseroles on a stovetop are slightly tricky, but it is possible. Place a portion of the casserole into a lidded pot with a tablespoon of water and a small amount of oil underneath the food. Keep it over a medium heat until it's warmed thoroughly. An oven is a great way to heat casseroles as it is usually best to warm food in the same method by which it was cooked. Put the casserole in the oven for 20 to 30 minutes at a medium temperature. For casseroles, the oven is the most ideal warming method, followed by the microwave and then the stovetop.

Soups

Soups that are prepared for freezing should be left slightly undercooked if they contain vegetables. Vegetables and some other ingredients, tend to lose their texture because of the moisture in the soup. They can become soggy and mushy, which is usually not a good texture. Be sure to leave space for expansion in whatever container you use to store the soup.

Before heating, thaw the soup overnight in the fridge. To heat portions of soup in the microwave, use a bowl that is big enough to allow a bit of space between the top of the soup and the top of the bowl. Microwave the soup for 30 seconds, then remove it and stir before putting it back for another 30 seconds. Repeat this process until the soup is very hot, then allow it to cool before eating.

Warming soup over a stovetop is much easier and much more effective. Bring the pot of soup to a boil, let it cool, and eat. Make sure that the pot has enough space between the top of the soup and the top of the pot to avoid any messes from boiling over. Heating soup in an oven is not ideal, and there's not really a method by which to do so.

Soups that have dairy ingredients should be warmed slowly to avoid curdling. Place them over a medium heat and stir as they warm. Add a bit of extra milk or cream while reheating to help freshen up dairy-based soups. For soups, the stovetop is the most ideal warming method, followed by the microwave and then the oven.

Breakfast

Breakfast is one of the easiest meals to prep for. Cooked eggs can maintain their quality even after 3 months of being frozen. This works best with eggs that are beaten before cooking. Scrambled eggs can be frozen in plastic bags or an airtight container. Egg patties or frittatas should be laid out flat on parchment paper and frozen until solid before it is placed in an airtight container or wrapped individually in plastic wrap or foil.

Eggs are one food that does not need to be thawed before being reheated. If you are using a microwave, cook the frozen eggs for 5 to 7 minutes. This will get rid of the extra water. To cook frozen eggs on the stovetop, place them in a frying pan over a medium heat and cook until warmed through. Warming frozen eggs in an oven will less likely leave them rubbery. Bake them for 12 to 15 minutes on a medium heat. Flip them halfway through if you'd like. For eggs, the oven is the most ideal warming method, followed by the microwave and then the stovetop.

Be sure to use the proper dishes for each warming method. Anything put in the microwave should be microwave-safe. If the container is plastic, ensure that it is BPA free and will not melt when warmed at a high temperature. For stovetop warming, be sure to use non-stick pans or use oil to grease the pan and avoid sticking. If you make a meal that contains different types of foods, know that each food will have a different ideal warming temperature and warming time. This does not necessarily mean that you need to separate them to warm your food. Stir the food while it cooks to make sure it warms evenly, and none of the ingredients get overcooked.

If your foods are not stored and reheated properly, the quality can be disappointing and discourage you from meal prep. To reap the full benefits of intermittent fasting, a healthy diet is important. Meal prepping can make following a healthy diet much easier and maintainable. Learning to meal prep correctly is an important component that will improve your lifestyle and help you reach your goals.

Chapter 9: 2 Week Meal Plan for Beginners

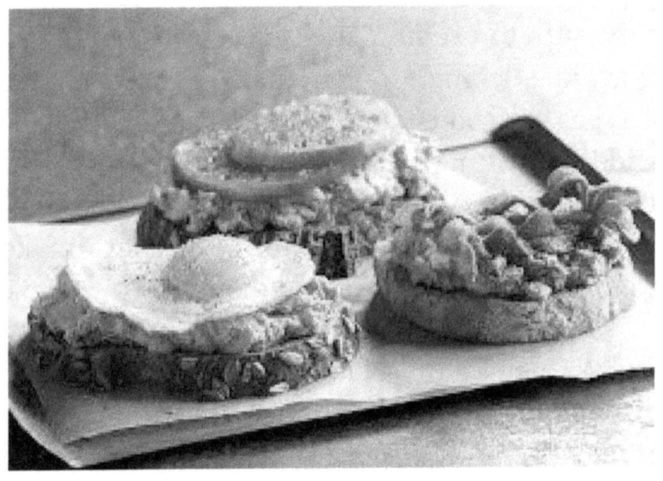

When starting your intermittent fasting journey, it's important to ease yourself into it. Starting out with a full 24-hour fast may leave your body feeling drained, and your motivation can fall away quickly. Doing too much too quickly can raise levels of cortisol in the body. Cortisol is a stress hormone that can make fasting harder by triggering the body to eat. It also hinders fat loss. To avoid excess stress, do not bite off more than you can chew. Gradually decrease the duration of your feeding window and increase the duration of your fasting window. Listen to your body and do what works for you. It's also always important to consult a doctor before implementing a fasting routine if you have any health issues that could be negatively affected.

For women, longer fasting periods can have negative effects on hormone levels that may cause hormonal issues and potentially damage the reproductive system. This limits the variety of intermittent fasting methods that women have to choose from.

For both men and women, the 5:2 diet is a great way to introduce fasting into your life. Because it never requires a full fast from calories, it can be less daunting to adjust to than other methods. By fasting on non-consecutive days and allowing calories during fasted periods, the body can adjust to having a caloric deficit, and you'll see results without a major shock to the system. Plus, you still get 5 days to go about your daily business as usual. Once you get used to fasting, you can change to a method that will best suit your lifestyle and the results you are looking for. To create a comprehensive meal plan that more readers can implement, we've used the 5:2 method. Here is an outline for a basic, 2-week meal plan to get you started on the 5:2 diet.

5:2 Diet Week 1	*Breakfast*	*Lunch*	*Dinner*	*Snack*
Monday	Normal	Normal	Normal	Normal
Tuesday	Normal	Normal	Normal	Normal
Wednesday	Restricted	Restricted	Restricted	Restricted
Thursday	Normal	Normal	Normal	Normal
Friday	Normal	Normal	Normal	Normal
Saturday	Restricted	Restricted	Restricted	Restricted
Sunday	Normal	Normal	Normal	Normal

5:2 Diet Week 2	*Breakfast*	*Lunch*	*Dinner*	*Snack*
Monday	Normal	Normal	Normal	Normal
Tuesday	Restricted	Restricted	Restricted	Restricted
Wednesday	Normal	Normal	Normal	Normal
Thursday	Normal	Normal	Normal	Normal
Friday	Restricted	Restricted	Restricted	Restricted
Saturday	Normal	Normal	Normal	Normal
Sunday	Normal	Normal	Normal	Normal

This outline shows a basic example of how to implement a 5:2 meal plan, but you can alter the schedule to fit your personal needs. As you can tell, this plan follows a "2 days on, 1 day off" schedule which causes the calorie-restricted days to fall at different parts of the week during the first and second weeks. If you want a more reliable routine, you can maintain the same fasted days every week. Be sure you are allowing at least 24 hours, if not more, between fasted days. By spacing the two calorie restricted days so that there are at least 24 fed hours in between, you give the body time to refuel before restricting again. Also, restricting on multiple days that are close together can increase the chances of binge eating on normal calorie days.

For optimal weight loss results, incorporate a healthy, balanced diet that will encourage fat burning and the presence the necessary amounts of key nutrients. On restricted days, make the most of the 500 to 600 calories your fasting routine allows. Include fruits, vegetables, and low-calorie proteins to keep your body properly fueled. The following meal plan is based on an approximate 2000 calorie diet on normal days and an approximate 500 to 600 calorie diet on restricted days. It will provide a few ideas on how to ration your calories and what foods to eat to help achieve the most effective weight loss. These meal suggestions do not take into account food allergies, diet restrictions, specific macronutrient ratios, or gut disorders, so alter the meals to fit your specific needs.

Week 1

Monday (normal calories):

      Breakfast- Raisin Bran Cereal (434 calories)

          *1.5 cups of 1% milk

          *1.5 cups of raisin bran cereal

      Lunch- Black Beans and Shrimp Quinoa Bowl (650 calories)

          *.75 cup quinoa

          *1 cup black beans, cooked with spices

          *.5 cup green pepper

          *.5 cup yellow onion

          *5 ounces shrimp, cooked with green pepper and onion

          *1 tablespoon olive oil to sauté

      Dinner- Salmon and Brussel Sprouts (592 calories)

          *1 cup brown rice

          *1 cup Brussel sprouts, roasted

          *1 tablespoon walnuts

          *5 ounces salmon

          *1 tablespoon olive oil for cooking

      Snack- 1 orange (62 calories)

Total: 1738 Calories

Tuesday (normal calories):

      Breakfast- Avocado Toast (402 calories)

          *.25 cup salsa

          *half an avocado, mashed

          *2 large eggs

          *1 slice whole-wheat toast

      Lunch- Salad with Chicken (500 calories)

          *.66 cup carrot, shredded

          *.5 cup cucumber, sliced

*8 cherry tomatoes

*5 ounce chicken breast

*3 cups spinach

*1 tablespoon olive oil

Dinner- Chicken and Asparagus with Quinoa (504 calories)

*12 pieces asparagus

*1 cup quinoa

*5 ounces chicken breast

Snack- Yogurt with Berries (239 calories)

*1 cup fat-free Greek yogurt

*20 blackberries

*1 cup strawberries, halved

*2 teaspoons honey

Total: 1645 Calories

Wednesday (restricted calories):

Breakfast- Spinach Omelet (160 calories)

* 2 medium eggs (140 calories)

*60 grams of spinach leaves (20 calories)

Lunch- 60 grams of Edamame beans (84 calories)

Dinner- Ginger, Apple, and Carrot Smoothie (107 calories)

*Ginger (0 calories)

*1 Apple (55 calories)

*1 Carrot (52 calories)

Snack- Banana (112 calories)

Total: 463 Calories

Thursday (normal calories):

Breakfast- Raisin Bran Cereal (434 calories)

*1.5 cups of 1% milk

*1.5 cups of raisin bran cereal

Lunch- Tuna and White Bean Salad over Spinach (498 calories)

*2 tablespoons sliced almonds

*2 tablespoons feta cheese

*.5 cup tomatoes

*.5 cup cucumber

*.66 can white beans, washed

*2.5 ounces canned tuna, drained

*2 cups spinach

Dinner- Black Beans and Shrimp Quinoa Bowl (650 calories)

*.75 cup quinoa

*1 cup black beans, cooked with spices

*.5 cup green pepper

*.5 cup yellow onion

*5 ounces shrimp, cooked with green pepper and onion

*1 tablespoon olive oil to sauté

Snack- Banana and Berries (160 calories)

*1 banana

*20 blackberries

Total: 1742 Calories

Friday (normal calories):

Breakfast- Ricotta and Pear (501 calories)

*1 cup ricotta cheese

*3 teaspoons peanut butter

*1 pear

Lunch- Salad with Chicken (500 calories)

*.66 cup carrot, shredded

*.5 cup cucumber, sliced

*8 cherry tomatoes

*5 ounce chicken breast

*3 cups spinach

*1 tablespoon olive oil
Dinner- Cajun Fish and Rice (620 calories)
*110 grams cream dory with seasoning
*.3 cup brown rice
*1 cup steamed mixed vegetables
Snack- Banana with Peanut Butter (235 calories)
*1 large banana
*1 tablespoon peanut butter
Total: 1856 Calories

Saturday (restricted calories):
Breakfast- Fruit and Yogurt (116 calories)
*1 apricot (17 calories)
*50 grams of raspberries (19 calories)
*50 grams of blackberries (20 calories)
*50 grams of strawberries (16 calories)
*3 tablespoons of fat-free Greek yogurt (24 calories)
*1 teaspoon of honey (20 calories)
Lunch- Asparagus and Boiled Egg (120 calories)
*5 pieces of asparagus (20 calories)
*1 large boiled egg (100 calories)
Dinner- Spinach and Turkey Breast (216 calories)
*1 cup of spinach, cooked (41 calories)
*125 grams of turkey breast steak (175 calories)
Snack- 20 Blackberries (48 calories)
Total: 500 Calories

Sunday (normal calories):
Breakfast- Raisin Bran Cereal (434 calories)
*1.5 cups of 1% milk
*1.5 cups of raisin bran cereal
Lunch- Chickpea and Veggie Salad (498 calories)
*1 tablespoon feta cheese

*2 tablespoons chopped walnuts

*.75 cups washed chickpeas

*.5 cups tomatoes

*.5 cups cucumbers

*2 cups spinach

Dinner- Chicken and Asparagus with Quinoa (504 calories)

*12 pieces asparagus

*1 cup quinoa

*5 ounces chicken breast

Snack- Ricotta and Pear (501 calories)

*1 cup ricotta cheese

*3 teaspoons peanut butter

*1 pear

Total: 1937 Calories

Week 2

Monday (normal calories):

Breakfast- Avocado Toast (402 calories)

*.25 cup salsa

*half an avocado, mashed

*2 large eggs

*1 slice whole-wheat toast

Lunch- Broccoli Shrimp Pasta Salad (297 calories)

*2 tablespoons red wine vinegar

*2 teaspoons olive oil

*1 tablespoon lemon juice

*1 teaspoon capers

*4 sun-dried tomatoes

*.5 cup broccoli, steamed

*.5 cup macaroni, boiled

*4 ounces shrimp
Dinner- Quesadillas (640 calories)
    *.25 cup sour cream
    *.5 cup shredded cheese
    *2 wheat tortillas
    *1 tablespoon lime juice
    *2 tablespoons olive oil
    *half of a roasted diced red onion
    *half of a roasted zucchini
    *half of a roasted green pepper
Snack- Hummus and Cucumber (119 calories)
    *4 tablespoons hummus
    *1 cup sliced cucumber
Total: 1458 Calories

Tuesday (restricted calories):
    Breakfast- Ginger, Apple, and Carrot Smoothie (107 calories)
        *Ginger (0 calories)
        *1 Apple (55 calories)
        *1 Carrot (52 calories)
    Lunch- Hummus and Veggies (175 calories)
        *sliced carrot, cucumber, and green pepper (52 calories)
        *40 grams hummus (123 calories)
    Dinner- Spinach and Turkey Breast (216 calories)
        *1 cup of spinach, cooked (41 calories)
        *125 grams of turkey breast steak (175 calories)
    Snack- 10 Pistachios (60 calories)
Total: 558 Calories

Wednesday (normal calories):

Breakfast- Raisin Bran Cereal (434 calories)

*1.5 cups of 1% milk

*1.5 cups of raisin bran cereal

Lunch- Chickpea and Veggie Salad (498 calories)

*1 tablespoon feta cheese

*2 tablespoons chopped walnuts

*.75 cups washed chickpeas

*.5 cups tomatoes

*.5 cups cucumbers

*2 cups spinach

Dinner- Salmon and Brussel Sprouts (592 calories)

*1 cup brown rice

*1 cup Brussel sprouts, roasted

*1 tablespoon walnuts

*5 ounces salmon

*1 tablespoon olive oil for cooking

Snack- Strawberry Toast (215 calories)

*8 strawberries, sliced

*1 slice wheat bread

*1 tablespoon peanut butter

Total: 1739 Calories

Thursday (normal calories):

Breakfast- Ricotta and Pear (501 calories)

*1 cup ricotta cheese

*3 teaspoons peanut butter

*1 pear

Lunch- Tuna and White Bean Salad over Spinach (498 calories)

        *2 tablespoons sliced almonds

        *2 tablespoons feta cheese

        *.5 cup tomatoes

        *.5 cup cucumber

        *.66 can white beans, washed

        *2.5 ounces canned tuna, drained

        *2 cups spinach

    Dinner- Cajun Fish and Rice (620 calories)

        *110 grams cream dory with seasoning

        *.3 cup brown rice

        *1 cup steamed mixed vegetables

    Snack- 4 Dates (264 calories)

Total: 1883 Calories

Friday (restricted calories):

    Breakfast- Spinach Omelet (160 calories)

        * 2 medium eggs (140 calories)

        *60 grams of spinach leaves (20 calories)

    Lunch- Beetroot Salad (125 calories)

        *60 grams spinach (29 calories)

        *30 grams of feta (83 calories)

        *50 grams of beetroot (13 calories)

        *lemon juice (0 calories)

    Dinner- Asparagus and Boiled Egg (120 calories)

        *5 pieces of asparagus (20 calories)

        *1 large boiled egg (100 calories)

    Snack- 60 grams Edamame (84 calories)

Total: 489 Calories

Saturday (normal calories):

Breakfast- Raisin Bran Cereal (434 calories)

*1.5 cups of 1% milk

*1.5 cups of raisin bran cereal

Lunch- Tuna and White Bean Salad over Spinach (498 calories)

*2 tablespoons sliced almonds

*2 tablespoons feta cheese

*.5 cup tomatoes

*.5 cup cucumber

*.66 can white beans, washed

*2.5 ounces canned tuna, drained

*2 cups spinach

Dinner- Quesadillas (640 calories)

*.25 cup sour cream

*.5 cup shredded cheese

*2 wheat tortillas

*1 tablespoon lime juice

*2 tablespoons olive oil

*half of a roasted diced red onion

*half of a roasted zucchini

*half of a roasted bell pepper

Snack- Strawberry Toast (215 calories)

*8 strawberries, sliced

*1 slice wheat bread

*1 tablespoon peanut butter

Total: 1787 Calories

Sunday (normal calories):

Breakfast- Avocado Toast (402 calories)

*.25 cup salsa

*half an avocado, mashed

*2 large eggs

*1 slice whole-wheat toast

Lunch- Chicken and Asparagus with Quinoa (504 calories)

*12 pieces asparagus

*1 cup quinoa

*5 ounces chicken breast

Dinner- Broccoli Shrimp Pasta Salad (297 calories)

*2 tablespoons red wine vinegar

*2 teaspoons olive oil

*1 tablespoon lemon juice

*1 teaspoon capers

*4 sun-dried tomatoes

*.5 cup broccoli, steamed

*.5 cup macaroni, boiled

*4 ounces shrimp

Snack- 4 dates (264 calories)

Total: 1467 Calories

Grocery List

Protein:

Chicken
Turkey Breast
Canned Tuna
Salmon
Cream Dory
Shrimp
Eggs

Vegetables and Beans:

Beetroot
Broccoli
Sun-Dried Tomatoes
Zucchini
Mixed Vegetables
Red Onion
Yellow Onion
Green Peppers
Brussel Sprouts
Carrots
Cucumbers
Tomatoes
Spinach
Asparagus
Edamame
Chickpeas
White Beans
Black Beans
Capers

Fruits:

Banana
Apple

Strawberries
Blackberries
Raspberries
Apricots
Pears
Avocados
Lemons
Limes
Dates
Oranges

Nuts:

Pistachios
Almonds
Walnuts

Pasta, Grains, and Bread:

Quinoa
Brown Rice
Macaroni
Whole-Wheat Bread
Whole-Wheat Tortillas

Other:

Feta
Sour Cream
Shredded Cheese
1 percent Milk
Fat-Free Greek Yogurt
Ricotta
Hummus
Honey
Ginger
Peanut Butter

Olive Oil
Raisin Bran Cereal
Salsa
Red Wine Vinegar

This meal plan is designed to give you enough variety that you do not get bored eating the same meals constantly while still allowing the option of batch cooking or eating leftovers. If you wish to simplify the meal plan for meal prep purposes, choose 2 to 3 types of protein to use over the two weeks and use the recipes that include your protein choices in place of the recipes that do not. All calorie values are estimates and may differ depending on the size or brand of the ingredients you use. Meal prepping once or twice a week will help you ensure that you stick to your healthy diet and gain the maximum benefits from intermittent fasting.

Conclusion

Thank for making it through to the end of *Intermittent Fasting: Guide for Women and Men.* We hope it was informative and it provided you with all the tools you need to achieve your weight loss goals, muscle gain goals, or even just improve your health.

See what all the historical hype is about for yourself by experiencing the benefits of fasting firsthand. The next step after reading this book is to figure out which method works for you and how you can begin incorporating intermittent fasting into your life! Take into account your physical health and the ways fasting can affect it and what you are trying to achieve through fasting. Some fasting routines are so simple to implement that you may find that you hardly notice the restriction. Apply the weight loss tips and tricks to see the fat melt away faster and follow the meal plan to see how a balanced, healthy diet can add to the benefits of your fast!

We hope that your experience with intermittent fasting brings you better health and satisfying maintainable weight loss. The benefits of fasting on your heart and brain can impact every aspect of your body. The better your body operates and the better you feel inside, the better your life will be. Improve your health, improve your happiness, and improve your existence!

Finally, if you found this book useful in any way, a review on Amazon is always appreciated!

Description

You've heard the hype about how people are seeing their fat disappear without changing what they eat, now you want to know what intermittent fasting is really about. This guide will give you all the information you need to get started and help you understand what's happening behind the scenes of those weight loss success stories.

This comprehensive guide will give you:
- A look into how fasting has been changing lives for thousands of years.
- An understanding of how intermittent fasting works.
- A deeper look at the abundant health benefits of fasting can inspire.
- A breakdown of all the major intermittent fasting methods and how to implement them.
- Tips on how to achieve major fat loss with fasting.
- Tips on how you can gain muscle even while your body is burning fat.
- Everything you need to know about using meal prep to meet your goals.
- BONUS: Two weeks 5:2 diet meal plan with a grocery list!

Intermittent fasting is praised by so many because it's not a diet, it's just an eating schedule. It's one of the simplest things you can do to improve your health on a cellular level while getting the results you want on the outside.

www.ingramcontent.com/pod-product-compliance
Lightning Source LLC
Chambersburg PA
CDIIW061507050706
48657CB00005B/1751